Stallside

MY LIFE WITH HORSES & OTHER CHARACTERS

Matt Eliott, DVM

Summer 2013

Stallside

MY LIFE WITH HORSES & OTHER CHARACTERS

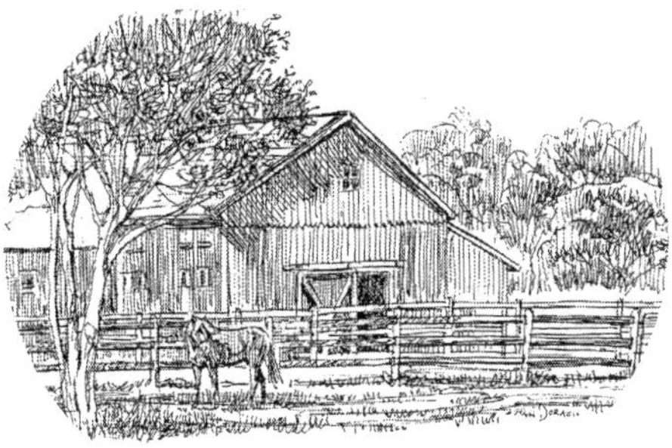

Matthew Eliott, DVM

Illustrations by Susan Dorazio

RiverHorse Press

First published in the United States of America in 2013 by
RiverHorse Press, North Salem, New York

Project Manager: Della R. Mancuso, Mancuso Associates Inc.
Creative Director: Mary Kornblum, CMYK Design Inc.
Cover and interior illustrations: Susan Dorazio
Editing: Rick Ball

ISBN: 978-0-615-81488-9

Printed and bound in the United States by
Worzalla, Stevens Point, Wisconsin

Contents

Introduction

I was born in South Africa, moved to the West Indies at the age of four. When I was eight I moved to New York City on a snowy winter's day and wouldn't see my dad again for fifteen years, until a week before he died. On the day I arrived in New York my life suddenly changed drastically, and it was a difficult transition. But time would pass and by the third grade I could tie my own tie, I wore a jacket to school, had already been to a lot of museums, and had a growing stash of comic books under my bed. By the sixth grade I was becoming a true city kid: I had a bus pass, took subways by myself, was getting good at skateboarding, and made futile and repeated protestations about having to attend dancing lessons after school on Wednesdays.

At the end of eighth grade I would have preferred to stay with my friends in the city, but the decision to attend a boarding school was not mine to make. Over the next four years, however, I would make new friends, and one in particular would quietly alter the direction of my life. On a visit to his house one weekend, I had a chance to talk with his dad, who sensed that I was struggling to find my way in life as perhaps he had when he was younger. He suggested my taking a year or so off after high school to "sort things out." My friend's dad lived in New York but was originally from Texas and had ties to the King Ranch in south Texas, which was trying to introduce into Australia a new breed of cattle known as Santa Gertrudis. "If you can find your way over there, you've got a job," he said. Less than a month after receiving a handshake and a diploma from the headmaster of my boarding school, I set foot on the gangplank of a freighter bound for Australia and wouldn't return to America for almost three years.

"Wonderfully difficult" would best describe the next year of my life, working on an enormous sheep and cattle ranch in Western Australia. The wildlife was extraordinary, the work arduous, and herding cattle and sheep on horseback for days at a time in the outback was an opportunity to gain perspective. A seed had been sown, but clarity of purpose does not come readily when one is in the late teens. I would backpack my way around Asia, Africa, and South America for a couple more years before hiring on as a "roughneck" on an oil rig outside El Paso, Texas. I needed the money, and when I quit it wasn't so much because of the precarious and clangorous conditions on the derrick floor, it was more of a quiet revelation that my dad would have wanted me to do more with my life. He had a degree in chemistry from UC Berkeley and was awarded a scholarship to obtain a PhD at a university in South Africa. He would have encouraged me to go to college, to learn how to learn, and to pursue a life's passion. Looking back, a common theme of my travels became apparent, my fascination with and love of animals, from the commonplace to the exotic. I decided I would go to college and pursue a degree in biology, and something to do with animals: cattle—or maybe horses.

My dad was absent from my life during this time, and it took me many years to articulate the purpose of my three-year "walkabout" of the world as being a search to find him in my life. As a veterinarian, years after he had died, I would find myself thinking about him on my way back from calls, driving along the Pacific Coast Highway. The absence of my dad from my life had been, at times, an equally dynamic inspirational force in seeking purpose and direction as his presence.

There were seventy-two of us in my graduating class from veterinary school, and our interests led us along diverse paths. A few wanted to be zoo vets, having an affinity for the lumbering, slithering, striped creatures. Many would work in mixed practices, taking on the care of cats and dogs in the morning and making farm calls in the afternoon. Some would work with just beef cattle and others only with dairy. There were those whose dream was to provide care for the likes of orcas, dolphins, and sea lions in the giant seaquariums.

"A chance to cut is a chance to cure" was the banner call of future surgeons. Others in my class wanted little to do with animals unless they were sectioned, stained, and presented on a microscope slide as a tissue specimen. These were the pathologists who unraveled the conundrums of viruses, bacteria, and protozoa. Those disturbed by the sight of blood seemed destined for radiology, where revelations about life were best seen on a viewing screen. The bright and brainy gravitated to the giant pharmaceutical companies, whose employees end their day at 5:00 P.M., never work weekends or get called out on emergencies, and enjoy paid vacations. I was not one of those.

I was the only one in my class who would choose to work exclusively with horses. Perhaps the rest of my class knew something I didn't; I preferred to think it was actually the other way around. The decision came easily. Horses seemed magical to me, and I felt moved to marvel whenever I was around them. It was serendipitous that horses also provided a forum for significant relationships to develop stallside. Friendship, laughter, sometimes a hug and occasional tear, all bring meaning to life.

I set up my first equine practice along the coastal hills of central California, having finished a two-year residency at the veterinary school at UC Davis. This part of California was big into cattle ranching and Quarter horses, a world where the gals grew up barrel racing, the guys team-penned or roped steers, and one of my first calls would be at a bucking-horse farm. The cowboys knew I appreciated their support, and the bond that grew us together was all about the horse. I didn't mind that, before making a call to me, they tried to treat their colicky horse with a pint of Jack Daniel's and a shot of brake fluid down the horse's ear. They never mentioned that I didn't own a pair of Levi's with a back pocket rimmed and faded from where a tin of Skoal smokeless resided. What mattered to them was if I could suture up a cow pony's barbed wire laceration and do a "right nice job" of it.

As you read through the stories in this book you will be introduced to an array of characters both equine (and some not) and human. Tiny and Tim were a couple of one-ton

Belgian draft horses owned by a farmer in California, where I had my practice. A few miles down the road was a dressage rider and trainer; nearby, an orchid grower had a barn full of miniature horses. Around the bend from him was Clifford's place—he raised mules. Further down the coast was the anxious owner of an Arabian horse gelding, a competitor in California's rigorous 100-mile endurance ride, the Tevis Cup. Past the vineyards of Fetzer was the foxhunter that rode with the Santa Ynez Valley Hounds. And of course, the cowboys.

It would be a few years in practice before I would pursue a different challenge, one almost as difficult as veterinary school: taking up the reins and swinging a leg over the saddle. Brushing dirt off the backside of my britches is what I seemed to do more than most, but I was persistent. Riding and competing with my horse has allowed me to see another dimension to veterinary medicine, the perspective of the horse owner. Being able to relate firsthand to the angst of noticing that one's horse doesn't finish breakfast or takes a lame step has given me an empathetic insight into how a horse owner feels waiting for the vet to pull into the driveway.

Somewhere along the way I began to jot things down here and there—fun stories, recollections of horses and their owners. I was asked to contribute a story to a newsletter in my hometown of North Salem, and then several more. The idea of collecting the stories into a book was partly the inspiration of my wife, Alexis. And without really planning to, I suddenly find myself an author. Writing was something I both enjoyed and grew up around. My mom was the author of several books, my stepdad was in the business of magazines and news; my grandfather wrote both a novel and a book of poems. My godmother, Nadine Gordimer, who still lives in South Africa, had her first book published when she was only fifteen years old. Her writing has long dealt with the moral and racial issues of the apartheid regime in South Africa, and her books would change much for the better in that part of the world.

Stallside is likely reminiscent of the tales any horse veterinarian might tell, though each one's experiences are unique and the path I have taken is my own—and so are the stories. I hope you will find as much pleasure and interest in reading them as I had in living through them and writing about them. Anyone involved with the magnificent and complicated creature that is the horse knows there is humor, challenge, reward, and humility in the lives of those privileged to have shared them with horses.

Matthew Eliott, DVM
North Salem, New York
July 2013

[ONE]

Ebb Tide

"HE'S GOT 'DIAHREAR' PRETTY BAD. What do ya think?" the cowboy asked me.

"Yup, I agree," I said as I moved Ranger's tail to the side and examined the smeared manure stains running down both hind legs.

Ranger was a working ranch horse and I remember him well because he was my first patient after I set up practice in the foothills along the central coast of California years ago.

"How long has this been going on?" I asked.

"Well, I know he ain't been doin' right for a couple of months now but the 'diahrear' just started up a couple of weeks ago I reckon," the cowboy responded.

"Let me have a listen on him," I said as I took out my stethoscope.

It was a typical summer day in June along the coastal hills of central California. It was 112°F and there wasn't a cloud in the sky. It would be several months before the winter rains came. The ground was hard, the grass was brown, and the beautiful live oak trees that grow along the coastal hills and canyons provided the only bit of shade to be found by the cattle.

The cattle ranch was owned by an Italian family who made their fortune mining quicksilver in the California coastal hills in the days when miners used mercury to recover gold. They had a cow-calf operation, meaning that the two-thousand-head herd of Black Angus cows were pastured out on the coastal foothills to produce calves for later sale. The ranchers also had eight or so horses they used to work the cattle, of which Ranger was one.

Ranger stood quietly as I passed my stethoscope over his chest, along his flanks, and under his belly. His heart rate was normal and his lungs sounded clear but there was something unusual about his gut sounds. In the background of the normal bubbles and gurgles was a swishing sound.

The cowboy had a plug of Skoal under his lower lip and just then gave a spit of the brown tobacco juice onto the dusty ground. He was rough bearded, lean, and missing half a finger off his right hand, a not too uncommon injury of many a team roper. After heading up a steer, the cowboy quickly goes to dally up his rope around the saddle horn but on occasion a finger gets caught in one of the turns just as the rope comes taut.

I could tell he was becoming impatient with me. Even though I was likely his age, I looked younger, probably too young in his mind to be a vet, and I wasn't even the regular vet for the ranch. I was inexperienced, just out of vet school, and we both knew the real reason I was called out: It was a compassionate gesture on the part of the ranch owners to make the new vet in town feel welcome.

"Do you mind hanging on to him a bit longer?" I asked. "I just need to listen a little more."

The cowboy's hat was sweat stained and he wore a short-sleeved red-and-white checkered Western shirt with faux pearl snaps. His belt buckle was big. It was ornate and of gold and silver, and I figured he probably won it in a rodeo. It had an engraved illustration of a cowboy chasing down a steer on a horse with a lasso. His denim jeans were faded, and silver Texas-star spurs were strapped onto his dust-covered boots.

I felt awkward, out of place, and I sensed that somehow the cowboy knew what I knew. I didn't grow up around cows or horses, wasn't born in Texas or Oklahoma, and would have gotten myself tangled up in a lariat in trying to sort out how to use one. I didn't know how to team rope, ride bulls, hadn't even been to a rodeo, much less won anything at one.

As I moved my stethoscope back to where I heard the swishing sound under Ranger's belly, it suddenly dawned on me what I was listening to. It was a familiar sound, one I had heard before but never with a stethoscope. It was the sound one hears when swimming underwater in the ocean as the waves recede from the shoreline. It was the sound of shifting sand.

"I'll be right back," I said excitedly and ran back to my truck to get a sleeve and a squirt bottle of lube. I slipped on the shoulder-length sleeve, squirted out some lube onto it, and pulled Ranger's tail to the side. Ranger's head came up as I slowly inserted my arm into his rectum up to my elbow. I could feel some manure but I could also feel a lot of grit.

"I think I know what the problem is," I said to the cowboy as I withdrew my arm and brought out a handful of mostly sand rather than manure. "Here, have a look," I said, showing the cowboy.

"Well, I reckon that'd be why he ain't been doin' right," the cowboy responded, spitting some more brown tobacco juice out onto the ground. It was clear that the cowboy wasn't nearly as impressed as I was excited by my diagnostic skills in uncovering the cause of Ranger's diarrhea and ain't-doin'-right condition the last several weeks.

"How much ya reckon he's got in there?" the cowboy asked.

"At least thirty pounds or so I would imagine," I answered, guessing more than really knowing. "We'll have to bring him in to the clinic where I can treat him for five or six days to get all that sand out," I explained.

"I'll have to check with the boss and see if that's what they wanna do. We'll let ya know in a day or so 'bout bringing him in," the cowboy said, spitting more brown tobacco juice onto the ground.

I got back in my truck and drove past the dusty livestock yards thinking about having seen my first patient as a horse vet out on my own, a cow pony on a cattle ranch in California. It was a small but rewarding step along an incongruous-seeming journey.

As I drove past the cows and their calves on either side of the road and crossed the cattle guard to leave the ranch, I thought about my past and suddenly recalled the name of a book written years ago. It was a book I actually never read, I only remembered the title. It was called *Stranger in a Strange Land*.

I GREW UP IN NEW YORK CITY. I wore a tie and jacket to school every day from first grade through boarding school, took dancing lessons at the Colony Club on Park Avenue, and lived in an apartment on Fifth Avenue.

The cowboy likely wouldn't have been impressed that by the time I was twelve years old I could cha-cha and fox-trot. I was a city kid and liked to skateboard the slated sidewalks outside the Guggenheim Museum and spend time at the Central Park Zoo. I played a lot of chess and was pretty good at squash by the time I was fourteen. I could take subways by myself by the time I was nine and had already been mugged several times by the time I was ten. I played stickball on East Eighty-First Street. First base was sometimes a parked Eldorado and third base was on occasion a Bonneville.

The cowboy would have smiled, however, had I told him that as a kid I loved to read a lot of Western comic books and that his heroes as a child may also have been mine. He too was likely left in longing by the stars of TV shows like *Gunsmoke*, *The Lone Ranger*, *The Adventures of Rin Tin Tin*, and *The Roy Rogers Show*, and it was even possible that *The Alamo* starring John Wayne was also the first movie that he saw as a kid.

I HAD A SIX-STALL HOSPITAL BARN to which was attached an exam room where I had a set of stocks, some lab equipment, and a couple of microscopes. There was also a round pen which I kept in grass where I could lay down horses for any number of short-term general anesthetic procedures. It wasn't much but it was a start.

Ranger was dropped off the following day. They never let me know he was coming. I just found him in a stall. He would be my first in-clinic patient and would stay while I treated him for sand colic. His medical history on the intake chart I filled out was abbreviated as "ADR"—ain't doin' right—and diarrhea. I smiled at the recollection of the cowboy's mispronunciation of the word diarrhea the day before. "Diahrear" was in fact more descriptive of where the problem was and I wondered why it wasn't spelled that way in the first place.

Ranger stayed for six days. I would pass a stomach tube twice a day and, using a stomach pump, administer a pound or so of a bran-like substance called psyllium mixed in about a gallon of water. I'd have to pump fast once I mixed the psyllium in with the water as it gums up quick once you get it wet. The consistency of wet psyllium rapidly becomes sticky like that of peanut butter, which is actually how it works to carry out the sand in a horse that's "sanded."

It didn't rain much in the part of California where I had my practice, even though we got twice as much rain as the aptly named town of Bakersfield which was further inland. The arid climate in that part of California, coupled with the fact that most horses live to eat and not the other way around, would make for a lot of sanded horses that I would see over the next many years.

Sand in a horse's belly could manifest itself in a number of ways depending upon how much sand they had in their gut.

Most horses with any significant accumulation of sand were depressed, lethargic, and carried a rough hair coat. Additionally, their owners would often complain of a soured behavioral change likely due to the low-grade abdominal pain associated with the irritating effects of the sand grating on the delicate gut lining.

The sore and inflamed gut of a sanded horse also usually resulted in weight loss. Some horses would have an accompanying diarrhea while others might present with an acute painful bellyache or colic. Other horses would develop intestinal stones, or enteroliths, some the size of pebbles or golf balls, which would pass in the manure, and others the size of a bowling ball, which would have to be removed surgically. I would eventually have quite a collection of green-colored, bowling-ball-size enteroliths around the clinic that I would use as doorstops and paperweights, souvenirs from sand colic surgeries.

"He's ready to go chase some cows now," I said to the cowboy when he returned in a week to pick up a much better feeling Ranger.

"So ya reckon he's ready to go back to work?" the cowboy responded as I led Ranger out of the stall and barn to the back of the gooseneck livestock trailer.

"I got rid of all the sand in his belly for now but you'll have to give him some of this medication for a couple of days every month to make sure he doesn't get into trouble again," I said handing him a container of the psyllium and some instructions.

As Ranger hopped in the back of the stock trailer, the cowboy handed me an envelope. "Boss said for me to leave this here check with you," he said.

"But I haven't sent him a bill yet," I responded.

"He said you'd be asking that. Jus' fill it out and send him a receipt be fine."

As the cowboy got in the pickup and turned on the ignition, a country radio station came on. I could see a tin of Skoal smokeless on the dust-covered dashboard, and as I turned to walk back to the barn, the cowboy stuck his head out the window and called out, "Wait jus' a sec. The boss reckons we might be seeing ya again."

{TWO}

"*Brutacaine*"

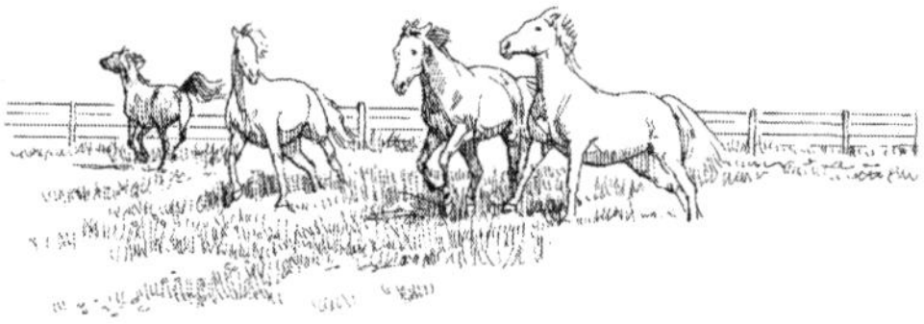

IT HAD ONLY BEEN A COUPLE OF MONTHS since I set up my practice, and easy street seemed just around the corner. I had gotten a call from a large Thoroughbred breeding farm in the area that wanted me to come do some work for them.

Ordinarily when the new guy in any business hangs out his shingle, he scavenges and hustles for work, often ending up working for clients and customers that no one else wants. I had gotten lucky. Landing a big account early on with a Thoroughbred breeder would allow me to bypass a lot of the startup trials and tribulations of being a new horse vet in town.

It was a call to vaccinate twenty or so horses. Each horse needed three different vaccines: rabies, a flu-rhino, and a 3-way, which is a combined vaccine of tetanus and a couple of viral strains of encephalitis.

Horse vets like getting called out to administer vaccines. It's called herd health and it's the bread, butter, and gravy part of any equine practice. Vaccinating horses is done during the morning or afternoon and is not something a vet needs to get out of bed in the middle of the night to do. It doesn't involve the back strain and sweat of picking up hooves and pulling shoes looking for stone bruises and foot abscesses, nor does it require a shoulder-length sleeve and an extra set of coveralls like the messy work of palping a bunch of mares for breeding. Lastly, it's not an adrenaline rush–filled experience like working with potentially dangerous stallions. It's a moneymaking cakewalk and something a vet can do without breaking a sweat.

Joe DiSalvo had been a real estate developer in Santa Clara up north. He had made a lot of money, retired out, and decided to get into the Thoroughbred breeding business. He bought a farm and some high-dollar brood mares and a stallion from Lexington's famous Thoroughbred auction house, Fasig-Tipton, and started breeding racehorses.

I pulled into the driveway outside the barn and hopped out of my truck. I was feeling excited. These were the kind of accounts it often takes a vet just starting out years of hustle to land. An added assurance was the fact that when I set up the appointment Joe had even mentioned that he would give me a check after we were done.

My first inkling that something was awry was the fact that the introductory handshake wasn't firm, and he was quick not to look me in the eye. He wore glasses, was short, balding, somewhat older, and in his shirt pocket was a copy of the *Daily Racing Form*, a trackside publication providing information on best bets, racehorse stats, and likely odds.

Despite being a horse owner he seemed unlike a horse person and somehow just not the type of guy you'd see with a carrot in his back pocket or someone who enjoyed making up a bran mash. Standing outside the stall door and smiling while listening to a horse munch on some hay just didn't seem like his thing.

"I'll meet you in the barn," I said to Joe as I grabbed the necessary vaccine vials from the fridge in my truck and a box of syringes.

As I headed into the barn, however, I didn't see any horses in the stalls. "They're out here," Joe said, holding a clipboard and waving me back outside the other end of the barn to where I could see some corrals.

There were about twenty of them, yearling colts and fillies milling around in a large corral, all with yellow numbered neck tags but no halters.

"Here they are," Joe said, handing me a halter and a lead rope. "I'll check 'em off as you get 'em done," he added, indicating his clipboard.

"Is there anyone else coming to give us a hand?" I asked as I looked back toward the barn, from which I hoped would appear a couple of barn workers to help catch up and hold the horses.

"Nope, just us," he replied, unconcerned.

When I opened the gate to the corral, it was as if I set off a near stampede. It was clear that little work had been done with these horses and I wondered if they were even halter broke.

"Have they had halters on 'em before?" I asked as I approached the mob of horses all huddled in one corner of the corral with their haunches turned toward me.

"It's been a while," Joe answered from the other side of the gate, looking down at his clipboard.

Catching them by managing to get a lead rope around their neck was the first step. Getting a halter on and dodging a sudden head toss was next. The fillies were rude and the colts rank. The ears would go back and they were quick to swing their haunches my way as I tried to approach from the side.

Once caught, I'd loop the free end of the lead rope around a fence post but without tying it off. Holding the lead rope with one hand would allow me a quick release if they panicked and pulled back, but it left me just my other hand to give the injections.

When it came time to administer the vaccines, I was forced to abandon near everything I had been taught about how to correctly administer an intramuscular injection. There wasn't enough time to *"remove the needle from the syringe, set the needle into the muscle, attach the syringe, aspirate, and slowly insert the medication."* It was a combined single action of jab and push.

"If you're going to give more than one vaccine, spread the injections around," is what I was taught. Administer one in the neck, another in the pectoral muscles, and another in a hind leg is the prescribed procedure. I successfully followed the recommendations of my Clinics professor on the first two yearlings and got kicked by the third when I tried to "set the needle" into a hind leg. The kick was high inside my thigh and I collapsed to the ground. "You okay?" Joe asked calmly from the other side of the corral. "Which one was that? Can you see his number?"

As I got back to my feet and hobbled back to get more vaccines from outside the corral, I recalled the insights of another Clinics professor: "*The ability to cow-kick is not species-specific; horses can do it too,*" and on minimizing the pain of being kicked it was emphasized that "*the closer you are to the hoof as it leaves the ground, the less it will hurt.*"

Insightful dispensations from the lecture hall, however, about how to minimize the pain are counterintuitive when a horse takes aim and the hoof leaves the ground. Instinct kicks in—hopefully before the horse has a chance to—and the response is one of moving away, not closer.

IT WAS SEVERAL HOURS LATER. I was exhausted, I ached, my coveralls were manure stained, and I would discover a couple more hoof prints on the inside of my leg that evening.

"Do I get a discount for having so many?" Joe asked before filling in the amount of the check.

"Brutacaine" was not something to be found in the rows of vials in the back cabinets of my truck and yet it was something I had to bring on most of my calls to Joe's farm. Over time there would be more hoof prints to be found on the inside of my legs, more manure-stained coveralls, and of course more requests for discounts.

THE CORNER OF EASY STREET AND WHISKEY was the address of my grandfather's winter house in Aiken, South Carolina, where he played a lot of polo. I would learn early on, however, as a horse vet that the easy street I had hoped to find wasn't just around the corner after all.

{THREE}

Gunsmoke and the Snakeskin Boots

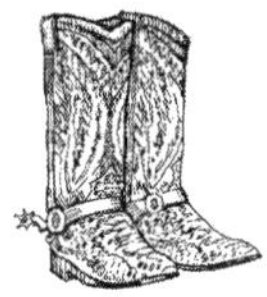

"A RATTLER GOT FESTUS. You better come quick," Larry said on the other end of the phone. "I'm twenty minutes away," I answered.

I turned down the driveway of Dodge City Ranch, pulled up in front of the barn, and saw Larry with a rattlesnake in one hand and Festus's lead rope in the other.

Festus was a six-year-old sorrel-colored Quarter horse gelding. He was a beefy rear-ended cutter and one of Larry's best horses.

"No doubt I guess you know a rattler got him," I said to Larry as I got out of my truck and looked at the dead rattlesnake he was holding.

"I was on my way out to the corral to catch up Festus and I saw the whole thing happen," Larry said. "I could hear that snake's rattlers buzzing from outside the corral, telling Festus don't you come no closer, but Festus jus' can't help himself none. He jus' has to go in sniffin' for a closer look, and all of a sudden like, that rattler gets him on the nose. I went and got my gun. Jus' can't have them rattlers comin' round the barn.

"You'd think Festus woulda' learned but I guess he ain't so smart about them rattlers. Same thing happened last year," Larry said. "A rattler come round the barn and Festus goes sniffin' some to check it out. I found the fang marks on his nose but it was a 'dry' bite and his head didn't swell none, but not this time: His head getting big in a hurry."

"Lemme have a look," I said and began to inspect the two fang marks on Festus's muzzle. Larry tossed the four-foot-long, large-scaled diamondback on the ground. "He's a big 'un. I'll get them eight rattles off his tail later and make myself a belt," Larry added.

Rattlesnakes appropriately belong to the genus *Crotalus*, a name derived from the Greek meaning "castanets." They are also a type of pit viper, with a heat-sensing pit organ located between the eye and the nostril on either side of the head, which allows them to "see" radiant heat. Night vision technology is nothing new for pit vipers. They have been using infrared stealth to detect and target warm-blooded prey in the dark of night since long before there were ever contracts between Lockheed and the military.

Festus's head was already the shape and size of a giant watermelon. Serum was starting to weep like honey from the skin around his muzzle, and the inflammatory edema in Festus's head was rapidly progressing to the point where his nostrils were beginning to swell shut.

The worst place for a horse to be bitten by a venomous snake is the head, and it's also the most common and it's usually on the muzzle. The concern is that the hemotoxic effects of the venom rapidly result in laryngeal edema and obstruction of the windpipe, causing the horse to suffocate. A bite to the leg wouldn't be nearly as worrisome, but that's not the part of the horse that goes sniffin' for trouble.

"Larry, I'll be right back," I said as I ran to my truck and grabbed a vial of the steroid dexamethasone, a sedative, some K-Y Jelly, and a couple of 35 cc syringe cases.

I slipped a needle into Festus's jugular vein and gave him a hefty IV dose of dexamethasone. "He's gonna have trouble breathing in a minute or two more," I said. "I'm gonna sedate him as well. He'll be less anxious about having difficulty breathing if he's sedated."

I gave Festus a triple IV cocktail of Rompun, Valium, and some Acepromazine. The sedation would also keep his heart rate down, slowing the spread of venom.

I cut off the end of the syringe cases, lubed them up with some K-Y, and gently inserted one up each nostril. The cylindrical syringe cases would keep his nostrils from collapsing shut. "If this ever happens again and I can't get here soon enough, you can cut off some garden hose and put a piece up each nostril.

"I'm not so sure what's gonna happen, Larry. That was a big rattler and packing a lot of venom. Festus is already starting to breathe pretty hard and his eyes are beginning to swell shut. I may have to cut a hole in his windpipe if the swelling moves to the back of his throat," I said.

"He's my best cutting horse. I jus' can't believe he ain't so smart about them snakes as he is about them cows," Larry said. "Is he gonna slough his muzzle?" Larry asked.

"That may be the least of it," I answered. "Depends on how much venom that rattler delivered. The venom destroys blood vessels, which causes internal bleeding. We'll start getting worried if he starts bleeding more than just a little out of both nostrils and if I have to go cuttin' a hole in his trachea so he can breathe."

Larry had a successful cutting-horse training barn and at any one time had five or six outside horses in for training. He also stood a couple of cutting-horse stallions, one of which was called Gunsmoke, a ten-year-old sorrel Quarter horse, and another by the name of Matt Dillon Dun It, a twelve-year-old, dun-colored Quarter horse. His best broodmare was a 12-year-old bay Quarter horse whose name was—as you might have already guessed—Miss Kitty. Festus, Larry's best cutting horse, was by Matt Dillon Dun It and out of Miss Kitty.

Cutting horses are almost always Quarter horses. They're quick, athletic, and a good one works with relish, savvy, and style. They call them "cutters" because their job in the event competition is to "cut out" a steer or heifer from a small group. As the separated steer or heifer tries to return to the herd, the rider loosens the reins—or in cutting-horse lingo "puts his hands down"—and leaves it entirely up to the horse to keep the steer or heifer separated. A contestant has just a couple of minutes to show the horse, and typically three steers or heifers are "cut" during a run.

It had been an hour or so since Festus had been bitten, and the hemotoxic effects of the rattler's venom were rapidly spreading, not subsiding. His eyes were swollen shut and his entire face was covered with beads of blood-tinged serum. The serosanguinous discharge from both nostrils was no longer a steady drip but was now becoming more of a steady flow. He was also beginning to drool ropey strands of saliva mixed with blood.

The viperous cocktail of tissue-destroying enzymes designed to rapidly break down the protein of the snake's prey as sort of a pre-digestive aid were doing just that. The phase of digestion involving the disintegration and dissolution of protein wasn't happening in the dark hollows of some digestive tract, it was something I could watch taking place right in front of me. Festus was getting worse, not better.

"We ain't gonna lose him, are we?" Larry asked.

"I'll be right back. I'm gonna give him another dose of dexamethasone," I said and dashed back to the truck.

I slipped the needle into Festus's jugular vein, attached the syringe, and pushed. I'd already given him more cortisone than I've had to give to any other horse going into shock, but the last dose of steroid didn't seem to be slowing down the swelling any.

"He ain't looking so good. Is there anything else we can do?" Larry asked.

"It's gonna be a wait-and-see deal," I told him. "We gotta keep him quiet and as long as he doesn't sound like he's snoring when he's breathing in, his windpipe isn't getting squeezed off and he should be okay. We'll know in an hour or so which way he's going."

I would see a lot of snakebit horses in California and almost all of them bitten by diamondbacks. Festus would be the most serious, however. I'd also end up treating a lot of bigheaded ranch dogs that found trouble coiled and rattling as well.

Ordinarily I'd stay and wait the hour or so after treating every rattler-bit horse or dog I saw to make sure they were going to be okay. I'd leave some antibiotics, a bit of "bute" as a pain reliever, and some more cortisone that they would be given orally over the next several days, and be out the driveway. I'd also often have a bit of time during the wait-and-see hour or so to tell the owners of my own experience with snakes.

IT WAS AT THE PASTEUR INSTITUTE IN THAILAND. The institute is actually a snake farm managed by the Red Cross and is the largest producer of antivenom serum in Asia. It's a part of the world where of the 400,000 or so people that are bitten by snakes every year, 20,000 die from the likes of the cobra, the banded krait, the deadly mangrove snake, and the saw-scaled viper.

Fortunately, the fastest land snake, the notoriously aggressive and deadly fifteen-foot-long black mamba, which travels with a third of its body above the ground striking in all directions, is found only in Africa.

A band of horses is well cared for at the Pasteur Institute. They are instrumental in the production of antivenom of some of the world's deadliest snakes. Once the venom is milked out from the snakes, small quantities of it are injected into the horses. The horses become increasingly resistant to the lethal venom as a result of the production of antibodies. Blood from the horses is then drawn and collected to obtain the serum from which the antivenom is harvested. The antivenom is then lyophilized—freeze-dried—placed in vials, shipped to hospitals, and made available to the likes of Asian rice farmers who work in cobra-dense wetland paddy fields.

The young Thai man whose job description on the snake farm included "venom extraction" told me to stand back just in case. It was a deadly spitting cobra that was dancing around in front of us with its neck flap or hood out and every so often lunging at the Thai man.

Skillfully, confidently, and quietly he grasped the snake's head and asked me to step closer and pass him the sterile collection receptacle. He pointed to the bulging saccular glands behind the snake's eyes and smiled. I watched the young man use the glass rim of the receptacle to pry open the mouth of the cobra and expose the two curved fangs. From out of the hollow fangs the venom flowed as the man squeezed the glandular sacs on the side of the snake's head. It was yellowish in color and translucent as it ran down the side of the glass vial. It looked like only a few milliliters, certainly no more than could fill a 3 cc syringe, but the Thai man spoke enough English to tell me this was enough venom to kill a thousand rabbits.

The snake farm had a small laboratory building where the venom was processed. There were some barns and corrals for the horses and there was also a large yard about one-third the size of a football field, caged and with a moat where several twelve-foot-long king cobras were gliding through the water. There were hundreds of snakes, all deadly, some slithering, some coiled, many swimming, and others mostly watching. Snakes smell with their tongues, and I could see the forked tongues flicking from a distance as we walked through the yard.

He pointed to a Siamese cobra and told me that after one bit him on the hand he had only six hours to live. The antivenom they produced on the farm saved his life, even though he sloughed the gangrenous finger a week later.

"HE DOESN'T SOUND GOOD. Whadda' we do now?" Larry asked. We both heard the beginnings of it, the heavy inspiratory snoring sound or "stertor" from Festus. "I'll be right back. He's not going to be able to breathe in another minute. We're gonna have to cut a hole in his windpipe," I said to Larry.

I should have clipped and prepped his neck just in case, I thought to myself as I ran back to the truck. Now there was only enough time to grab a vial of local anesthetic, some gauze pads, some disinfect, and a scalpel blade.

"He's gonna bleed some. You ready, Larry?" I said after having injected 10 cc of local anesthetic into the middle of Festus's neck.

"I don't care none about any blood but you better hurry, he doesn't sound good," Larry said.

I knelt down in front of Festus with a scalpel blade. "Peel the blister pack off and pass this to me when I ask for it," I said, handing Larry the *J*-shaped tracheostomy tube.

If you turn the letter *J* upside down, the hook at the bottom of the letter is that part of the tracheostomy tube that sticks out of the horse's neck. The longer stem portion of the letter is inserted into and down the trachea a couple of inches.

There wasn't much time. The stertor or snoring sound was becoming louder. Festus was now all but gasping for air as the inflammatory edema was swelling his airway shut. I quickly made a five-inch up-and-down longitudinal incision through the skin in Festus's neck, separated out the neck muscles, and located his trachea. A quick transverse incision between two of the tracheal rings was all that remained. "All right, Larry, lemme have it," I said. "We're in." The relief was almost immediate. The stertor stopped and Festus could breathe.

"Well, I ain't never seen that done before," Larry commented with a relieved smile.

"Well, I never had to do one before," I said.

"It's a good thing you didn't tell me that earlier. I was already shaking in my boots thinking I was gonna lose Festus."

It would be a bit of a long afternoon, a vigil that would extend into the night and the following couple of days.

"Can you stay with Festus tonight and run the rest of the fluids to him?" I asked Larry.

"Yup, sure can do. I'll just throw a sleeping bag in the back of the pickup and park outside his stall.

When you reckon he'll be able to eat or drink some?"

"Maybe a couple days, maybe longer. He's got to be able to swallow before he can eat or drink anything. He'll choke if he can't swallow, and right now he can't breathe without that tube in his windpipe," I answered as I finished throwing in a couple of whip stitches around the catheter in Festus's jugular vein. "In the meantime, we'll just keep running fluids to him. He's probably gonna drop a couple hundred pounds and skinny up some before he's really on the mend.

"Larry, can you rig something up in his stall so we can hang the fluids?" I asked as I got the IV lines ready to begin running some Ringer's solution to Festus.

Larry rounded up some baling twine and set up a simple pulley system over one of the crossbeams in a stall so we could raise and lower the five-liter bags of solution.

Festus would need thirty liters—almost eight gallons—of IV fluids daily before he was finally able to sip some water on his own three days later. He would also drop two hundred pounds of body weight before he could go back to eating hay.

"How's he gonna eat?" Larry asked.

"Like I told ya, he can't eat if he can't swallow, but here's how we'll kinda know when he's ready," I responded, taking my hand and covering the opening of the tracheostomy tube in Festus's neck. The snoring sound was immediate on the next breath that Festus tried to take. "When you can cover the tube and he doesn't make that sound, the swelling is down in his throat so that he can eat, drink, and breathe on his own.

"It's gonna take a week for his head to come down, and in the meantime you're gonna have to feed him like he busted his jaw," I told Larry. "Make him an alfalfa soup slurry or gruel, something he can sip, not chew, at least until his head has come back to size," I added.

Festus would slough a skin patch off his muzzle where he got bit the size of a pancake. The gangrenous skin blackened up, turned leather-like, and just fell off. We were able to pull both the tracheostomy tube and the IV catheter but not until the third day, when Festus was finally able to sip both water and a porridgy mix of soaked hay pellets. He did indeed skinny up some before the facial edema had subsided and he could chew on his own.

A couple of months later Larry called asking me to come to a barbecue he was having that Saturday afternoon. Larry had become both a friend and a good client, and of course I was curious how Festus was getting on.

I pulled into the driveway of Dodge City Ranch smiling and thinking of all the *Gunsmoke* characters Larry had as horses. I had gotten there a bit early, wanting to see Festus, and was met by Larry coming out of the barn. "Hey, Larry, how ya been?" I asked.

"Real good," he responded. "I was hoping you might be here a bit early. I got myself a new cutting horse."

"But what about Festus? He's all right, isn't he?" I asked.

"Oh sure, he's fine. C'mon in, he's right here."

Festus was indeed looking good. The skin over his

muzzle had grown back and he was looking fit and back to cuttin' cows.

"I found me a horse out of Miss Kitty that she foaled out a year before I bought her," Larry said excitedly.

"Well, let's have a look," I said. I followed Larry out the barn to a corral.

"Yup, when I found out he was a half-brother to Festus, I jus' had to have him and even changed his name to Chester," Larry commented as we stood outside the corral.

"So Matt Dillon didn't actually do it this time?" I asked jokingly.

"Nope, not this time," Larry replied. "Chester is out of Miss Kitty but by another dun-colored stallion."

"What's the stallion's name?" I asked.

"Dillon Dun it Again," Larry answered with a smile.

"He's a good-looker, Larry. Can he cut pretty good?" I asked.

"Almost near as good as Festus. He's smart and he likes chasing cows," Larry said.

LARRY WOULD BE KIND IN HELPING me grow my practice in California. It was mostly other cutters that were there at the barbecue, some of which would eventually become clients.

After the barbecue was over Larry and I pulled up some hay bales to have another beer outside Chester's corral.

"Yup, he was a big 'un," Larry said.

"What do you mean?" I asked.

Larry stretched out his legs and clicked his cowboy boots together. "That there's the real McCoy. Had 'em made custom," he said. I smiled as I recognized the snakeskin-covered cowboy boots. They were made from the large-scaled rattler skin of a diamondback.

{FOUR}

From Jamaica to Manhattan

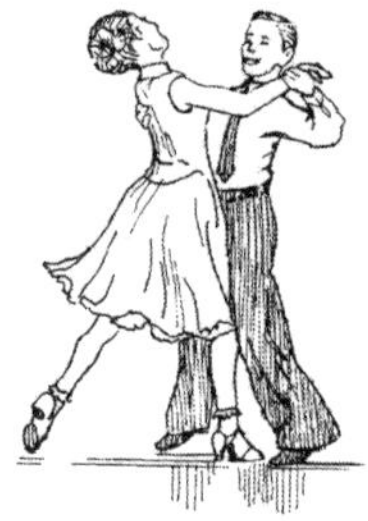

MY DAD WAS FROM CALIFORNIA. He grew up in the Buttermilks along the eastern foothills of the Sierra Nevada near Bishop. There are some pretty amazing rock formations in that part of the world, which I think in part is why he went to Berkeley to become a geologist.

My mom, however, was everything New York. She was a debutante: sophisticated, social, and beautiful. She turned down a scholarship at Radcliffe to travel the world, which is how she came to meet my dad.

The *California* was the name of the schooner my dad and some of his friends bought together. They sailed around the world for close on five years, and when they ran out of money in Southeast Asia, my mom was there in Bangkok to help them settle up on some bills and buy new sails, but only if they took her on as part of the crew.

My mom would write a book about the time she spent on the *California* called *Give Me the World*. I remember looking through the photos in her book when I was a kid. They sailed through the South Pacific long before there were hotels in places like the Nicobar and Solomon Islands. There were photos of the Dani tribe members from New Guinea with boar tusks through their noses and headdresses made from the feathers of Birds of Paradise. There was even a picture of a woman in a village outside Papua, New Guinea, breastfeeding a pig.

I was born in South Africa and we moved to the West Indies when I was four. My sister was born in a Kingston hospital when I was eight. The floors of the hospital were wooden and the patients' rooms opened up onto a courtyard where goats would graze. It was a time when ether was used as a general anesthetic, and I had my tonsils taken out that year. It was also a time when, if you got sick as a kid, doctors still made house calls. Unfortunately, however, from out of Dr. Shoemaker's black bag came the uniform curative for kids who weren't feeling well: an enema.

I was raised by black nannies, and Roy the gardener took me to school every day on his bicycle. Roy the gardener used a machete to cut off the tops of coconuts. We both liked them when they were green, not brown, when the "copra," the thin, white, sweet flesh inside was still soft and easy to scoop. We would share the milk inside and afterwards he would use his machete again to split open the nut and give me part of the husk as a spoon.

The cook made sure I had my daily spoonful of cod liver oil. I watched the cook once cut off the head of a chicken that we were going to eat that night. She didn't mind. She was the cook.

I ate a lot of ackee, saltfish, and dumplings. Curried goat was for special occasions and mangoes, jackfruit, and pawpaw (Jamaicans and kids prefer the name pawpaw rather than papaya) were what we ate for breakfast.

Mongooses lived in the tall grass behind our house. I would see them during the day. The cook didn't like them because on occasion they would break into the hen house and kill a chicken. The *Jungle Book* story of Rikki-Tikki-Tavi by Rudyard Kipling, however, was read to me when I was young, and even though Jamaica doesn't have any poisonous snakes, I liked knowing that mongooses lived near our house. We had lots of pearl guinea fowl, the dark gray ones with white dots throughout their plumage. They were pretty. They were also very noisy but my mother told me they ate lots of bugs, including bees and wasps.

Treasure Beach is along the south coast of Jamaica, and it's where we went almost every Sunday. It's where I learned to swim. The waves are big and as we waded out to where the waves would crash, my dad would hold my hand and together we would hold our breath and go under the water and let the waves pass above us. After coming back from the beach we made ice cream using a wooden bucket hand-crank ice cream maker.

Sugarcane is the world's largest crop, not rice, and they grow a lot of it in Jamaica. Whenever we visited Kingston my dad would stop and buy me a glass of freshly squeezed sugarcane juice with ice from the street vendors.

A tuppence could buy a Creamsicle, and the icebox was just that. Sawdust-covered blocks of ice were delivered every week by a mule-drawn wagon. When the men were done unloading the ice, they would let me ride on their wagon a ways up the road and then I would thank them, hop off, and run back home.

We poled down the Brae River once on a bamboo raft

from which we could jump off and swim in the Luminous Lagoon, where the river meets the Caribbean Sea and where a rare phosphorescent microbe lives. It's a near magical place for a kid, because swimming in the water causes the water to luminesce.

My dad was tall, handsome, and had blond hair and blue eyes. He could play the guitar, draw cartoons, and write in Chinese. He smoked a pipe and had a PhD in geology and a fishing business out of Kingston. The shallow waters and cays off the south coast of Jamaica provided good fishing for mackerel. I caught a barracuda once when he took me out on his boat and he had to help me reel it in. His other business was run out of a twin-engine Cessna, dropping silver iodide into clouds to make rain. He used to let me hold on to the yoke or control column when we were above the clouds and tell me I was actually flying the plane.

IT WAS SNOWING THE DAY WE MOVED TO NEW YORK CITY. We moved into an apartment on Fifth Avenue. My dad stayed in Jamaica and I wouldn't see him again until fifteen years later, a week before he died.

The next many years of my life would be very different, and the transition was difficult for me. My mother had returned with her children to her roots as an author and socialite in New York City. For me, however, this would be a stretch of time in my life where I would struggle.

I felt uprooted and certainly not in any way returning to a place of roots. My dad, my nannies, the cook, and Roy, the people who grew me up as a child, were no longer there. Kids are resilient, however, and the sounds of sirens, jackhammers, subways, and traffic horns would become integrated into my new life.

I tied a tie and wore a blue blazer to school every day. I took the subways and buses by myself before I turned ten and once even took the IRT Lexington Avenue Line subway all the way down to Canal Street in Chinatown to buy firecrackers. I sat on a park bench by myself and waited until a Chinese man came and asked me what I wanted. He came back with a brown bag and I gave him some money. When I was ten, I got mugged by three Puerto Rican girls. They took my bicycle.

I learned to skateboard, went to a lot of museums, and could shop by myself at Brooks Brothers by the time I was twelve. My best friend and I played a lot of chess.

I read a lot of comic books and secretly hoped I would one day wake up as Carter Slade, the mysterious Western hero known as the Ghost Rider. He rode a white horse named Banshee and his all-white costume, including a face mask, cape, and white hat, magically glowed.

I wore a gray suit to school every Wednesday for three years. Dancing lessons were on Wednesday afternoons at either the Colony Club on Park Avenue or the Hotel Pierre on Fifth Avenue. I went to a lot of junior cotillions at the Waldorf-Astoria and the Plaza Hotel. My mother relied a lot on the *Social Register*, a blue-blood directory of sorts from which she decided who should and shouldn't be my friends. Her own friends were artsy and different and the name of a cousin who lived in Scotland was the Dowager Lady Eliot of Stobs. Philip Glass once played the piano as Allen Ginsberg read his poetry in our living room.

When I was thirteen my mom took me to a boarding school, and although I would come home for vacations, the only time she came to see me was when I graduated four years later.

The summer I turned eighteen I booked passage on a freighter bound for Australia and left New York.

{FIVE}

Gonad the Barbarian

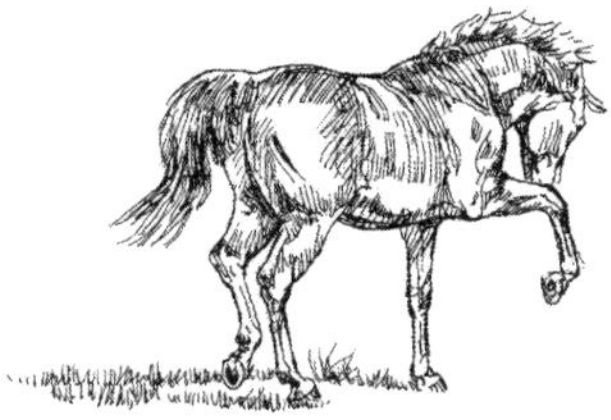

IT WAS A COOL MORNING IN OCTOBER along the coastal hills of central California. I was standing in the paddock behind Jack Reed's barn next to a three-year-old stallion I was about to geld. I had just given the stallion an IV triple cocktail of Rompun, Valium, and Torbugesic and was waiting for it to take effect before giving him the IV ketamine I had drawn up.

The IV triple cocktail and ketamine to follow is how most horses are put under general anesthesia for any number of short-term procedures. A vet has about twenty minutes to do what needs to get done before the horse comes out of the anesthesia.

I had Jack hang on to the lead rope as we both waited and watched. In less than a minute the stallion started to get a bit "sleepy-eyed" and hang his head. "He's starting to look pretty wobbly, Doc," Jack said.

"Yup, he's just about ready," I replied as I took out the

12 cc syringe of ketamine from my pocket.

Jack and I had been through this several times. He had been breeding and racing Quarter horses for almost thirty years and had a keen sense of what it took to breed a fast horse that would stay sound during its racing career. He kept the colts intact that he felt had the talent and speed to race and gelded the rest.

Running Quarter horses do just that. They're sprinters and can run a quarter mile faster than any other breed of horse. A beefy rear-ended Quarter horse can cut loose out of the starting gate like a rifle shot and clock out at 45 mph at the end of a quarter mile. The lean and catlike Thoroughbred tops out at only 30 mph but, like a marathon runner from Kenya, can go the distance that a Quarter horse never could.

"So why'd you wait so long on this one?" I asked as I bent down to cast a glance at what was impressively to be found between the stallion's hind legs. My eyes widened as I noted that each testicle was the size of a small grapefruit.

"You know, Doc, he's pretty quick and I'd thought he'd be a winner. But he's small footed and I couldn't keep him sound enough to keep running him," Jack replied.

"Well, he may be small footed but he made up for it elsewhere," I said, still staring at the job ahead of me.

"Yeah, he's 'Big and Tall' in that department all right," Jack said. "You don't think that's going to make it any more difficult to geld him, do you?"

"Not to worry," I told him. "We may need to keep him down a bit longer so he doesn't bleed so much when he gets up," I added.

"Whatever it takes, Doc. We just gotta get him cut. He'll make someone a real nice trail horse as a gelding and besides, I couldn't wait any longer. He was getting sort of rank."

Castrating or gelding a stallion is about as close as a horse vet gets to doing brain surgery. Macho is the sometimes stuff of Hollywood film characters like Conan the Barbarian. Testosterone, however, is responsible for the fact that stallions have the potential for starring in their own feature film version: *Gonad the Barbarian.*

A "rank" stallion is snaky, catlike, and quick to hurt you. "Vicious" might describe best what's on the other end of the lead rope of a rank twelve hundred pounds of testosterone. They can be incredibly quick to strike with a front foot and lightning fast with a hind leg. Their necks can be Herculean and their jaws powerful. In a catlike moment they can pick you up with their teeth, fling you across the stall, pin you down, and grab your throat.

"He's looking like he's starting to sway in the breeze, Doc," Jack said with a chuckle.

"I agree, he's looking pretty drifty," I remarked. I held off the stallion's jugular vein and slipped the 19-gauge, inch-and-a-half needle into his vein. I waited for the flash of blood to appear in the hub of the needle, then attached the syringe of ketamine and pushed. I withdrew the needle, capped it with the needle guard, and hoped that was all I'd need to give him.

"All right, here we go. I'll take him now, Jack," I said as I grasped the lead rope. "Can you bring that saddle pad and my long rope over?" I asked.

"Be right back," he replied.

The stallion's legs slowly buckled out from underneath him. I held tight on to the lead rope as he fell, so he wouldn't smack his head against the ground, then placed the Navajo saddle pad that Jack had returned with under the stallion's head. I reached into the back pocket of my coveralls and removed a blue hand towel which I then placed over the stallion's eyes.

I would have about twenty minutes. I made a slipknot out of one end of the thirty-foot cotton rope and placed it around the pastern of the hind leg that was down. "Okay, Jack, grab his tail and lift," I said as I pulled the rope under the stallion's haunches and figure-eighted the free end of the rope around the hocks and pastern of the hind leg that was up. I handed the cotton rope off to Jack and said, "Okay, he's all yours. Get the rope behind your back and lean into it so that he rolls up on his back." The front end of the stallion was on his side but his hind legs were up and spread apart.

I quickly brought my surgical pack over and knelt between the stallion's hind legs. I wiped down the scrotal area with several handfuls of water-soaked cotton and betadine disinfect and put on a pair of surgical gloves. "Jack, here we go," I said. I opened the silver pouch containing a No. 8 scalpel blade and attached the blade to the scalpel handle.

I squeezed with one hand the neck of the scrotum, forcing one of the testicles taut against the scrotal skin. With the scalpel in my other hand, I made a six-inch incision through both the skin and the connective tissue layer surrounding the testicle. "He's a whopper!" I said to Jack as the testicle popped out of the scrotal sac. I could feel the beads of sweat forming on my forehead as I pulled on the now-exposed testicle to get at the attached spermatic cord.

The spermatic cord is just that. It's a cord-like structure attached to the testicle that contains a good-size artery, vein, nerves, and the vas deferens. The vas deferens is a tubular structure that connects the epididymis of the testicle with the male urethra. It's the piece of anatomy that transports sperm and it's the structure that gets snipped when a guy has a vasectomy.

The spermatic cord also contains a substantial strap of muscle called the cremaster muscle. It's the "up and down" muscle that allows the testicles to descend on a hot day and to rise back up toward the belly on a cold day. In a three-year-old stallion this muscle can be surprisingly well developed and present a bit of a tug-of-war contest with a veterinarian.

"He's pulling back pretty good," I said to Jack as I stripped the fat off the cord with a handful of gauze pads.

"I don't blame him. I'd put up a fight too," Jack said.

Using a hefty bit of traction, I managed to bring enough of the spermatic cord out to where I could get the emasculators in place.

"Okay, Jack, hang on. This may wake him up a bit," I said. I positioned the stainless steel, double-bladed, crush-and-cut emasculators around the spermatic cord. With both hands and all my strength I was just barely able to squeeze the handles shut. The jaws of the emasculators made a crunching sound that even Jack heard as he stood behind me still leaning into the rope.

"I tell ya, Doc, that always sounds so final," Jack said.

The German-made emasculators I was using were the best that money could buy. As the handles were squeezed shut, the jaws would close around the spermatic cord. The first blade would crush the cord and its blood vessels and the second would cut.

"I'm gonna have to leave these on for a good two

minutes so he doesn't bleed any," I said to Jack as I glanced at my watch. The stallion had been out for just over six minutes and the IV general anesthesia I gave him should have kept him down for another fifteen minutes or so.

I was feeling a sense of relief at being halfway done when all of a sudden the stallion's head came up and his back legs gave a tug against the rope. "Doc, he's coming out of it!" Jack shouted in a panic.

I scrambled to stand up and get out from between the stallion's hind legs, leaving the emasculators in place. "Jack, drop the rope and lay on his neck. He'll be trying to stand if he can swing his head up." Jack did just that. He dropped the rope and laid his body across the stallion's neck. "Don't let him get up, I gotta get more drugs," I said as I sprinted toward my truck.

If you have ever seen a horse that was lying on its side get to its feet, it swings its head up first and the rest follows. If you can somehow body-block the horse's ability to swing its head up off the ground, you can keep it from standing up. Jack was lying with all his weight across the stallion's neck and head. Had it not been for the fact that the stallion was still groggy from the anesthesia, the stallion would have flipped Jack like a rag doll off to the side.

I ran back to the truck and grabbed the vials of Rompun and ketamine, a 20 cc syringe, and a needle. Frantically attaching needle to syringe, I withdrew both medications and dashed back to Jack, who was lying across the stallion's neck in a sweat, struggling not to let it stand.

I knelt down beside Jack. "I can't believe it, Jack. He was only down six minutes," I said as I slipped a needle into the stallion's jugular vein, attached the syringe, and pushed.

"You guys obviously didn't take the same pharmacology

class. What happened?" Jack humorously remarked.

My heart was racing. I flashed back to a time when a stallion came out from the anesthesia I had given him much too soon. . .

EVERY VETERINARIAN HAS A TALE THEY WOULD RATHER NOT SHARE, a milestone event that brings them to their knees, and what follows was mine.

I had been asked by a horse owner to geld their ten-year-old stallion behind the barn, and I agreed. Had wisdom prevailed, I would have declined and referred the owner and their older stallion to a veterinary hospital where, in the event of any surgical complications, additional veterinarians and staff would have been available.

I knew at the time that attempting to geld an older stallion would be much more of a surgical and anesthetic challenge than a yearling colt. I also knew that the blood vessels were more established and that I would have to extend the downtime by using additional anesthetics.

The precept of the Hippocratic oath admonishing physicians and veterinarians alike to "do the patient no harm" seemed an all too obvious, if not a ridiculous given. I was a couple of years out of veterinary school and I was cocky, presumptuous, and better judgment was eclipsed by a lack of humility.

I gave the ten-year-old stallion I was about to geld the triple IV cocktail I later gave to Jack's stallion. I had also given him an additional IV anesthetic called thiopental, a type of barbiturate, to extend the downtime, knowing that there would be a tendency to bleed if he tried to stand too early.

The castration procedure itself was uneventful. What I

didn't take into account, however, was the unanticipated stormy recovery that the stallion would experience coming out of the anesthesia. After the surgery, he should have lain quietly on the ground for half an hour or so, burning off the anesthetic meds I had used. But he didn't.

After only fifteen minutes of being down, the horse suddenly leapt to his feet. Still in an anesthetic delirium, he staggered a few steps then fell.

He repeatedly fell and scrambled to his feet only to careen about and fall again and again. Unsuccessfully, I tried to steady him whenever he got back to his feet. The horse's intestines prolapsed through its inguinal rings and out through the scrotal incision.

By the time the horse finally stood still it was too late. The calm at the end of the storm was calamitous. The horse's hind feet were surrounded by twenty feet of his own intestines. There was nothing to be done but to draw up one last injection. I walked back to the truck shaking, slid open the back cabinet, and reached for the vial of euthanasia solution.

Remarkably, the horse owner was understanding if not sympathetic. I remember now, twenty-five years later, as if it were yesterday driving out the driveway and pulling over to the side of the road after a mile or so. Trembling and with tears in my eyes, all I could think was: "What had I done?"

"JACK, I THINK WE'RE GOOD. Grab the rope and pull his hind legs up," I said as I put on another pair of sterile gloves. I knelt back down between the stallion's hind legs and squeezed the neck of the scrotum, forcing the remaining testicle taut against the scrotal skin.

"Here we go, Jack," I said and made a second six-inch

incision through the scrotal skin and connective tissue.

"Yup, he's *grande*, all right," Jack said as he peered over my shoulder and watched the remaining testicle pop out. I reached for the emasculators again, placed the jaws around the spermatic cord, and with both hands squeezed the handles shut. The crunching sound reminded me of a funny story.

I WORKED WITH A GAL VET ON OCCASION, and every so often we'd geld a couple of colts together. She enjoyed catching me off guard with her quick and sometimes barbed sense of humor. On one occasion, as she squeezed the handles of the emasculators shut, causing the sound of the crush to be heard, "Said you'd call" is what she said under her breath, just loud enough for me to hear. She didn't look up but I could see that she was smiling.

AFTER FIFTEEN MINUTES OR SO, the colt got to his feet. "Jack, you know the post-op routine," I said. "Rest him today but then begin trotting him lightly twice a day for the next couple of weeks. That'll keep the swelling down." I packed up my gear and watched as Jack led his new gelding back to the barn.

It was a month or so later that I found a package on my desk at the veterinary office. It was from Jack Reed. "Hmmm," I thought to myself as I opened it up. There was a T-shirt and a note that simply said "Thanks, Doc, he's a different horse." I held up the T-shirt, the front of which read: "Stallions are from Venus, Mares are from Mars, and Geldings are from Heaven."

{SIX}

Adjusting Henry

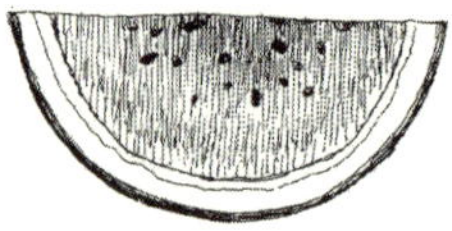

HENRY WAS A HUGELY SWEET, DAPPLE-GRAY PERCHERON draft horse stallion I bought from an old California dairy farmer. His feet were enormous, his body thick and well rounded, not at all angular like a Thoroughbred, and his disposition, like most draft horses, kind to the point of almost being timid. He enjoyed eating watermelon, and I recall many times smiling as I listened to him munching on the juicy rinds, watching the watermelon juice run down his chin, his eyes glassy and trancelike, clearly savoring one of life's simple pleasures.

Henry's foals, especially the Thoroughbred-cross offspring, were popular with the local foxhunt. The Thoroughbred-draft cross was a less complicated horse than the Thoroughbred and would tend to stay sound longer, as the dry, hard footing of California was unforgiving on a small-footed horse. The quiet and willing disposition of the draft cross resulted in a horse that was well mannered when in company with other horses, as well as around the hounds.

The breeding operation I had going with Henry turned out to be somewhat of a growing side business in addition to my veterinary practice. I kept the stud fee low at 250 dollars and as an added draw I included a live-foal guarantee. It worked out quite well; the mare owners for the most part lived locally so I often ended up providing the routine veterinary care for the mares during their pregnancy and for their foals after they were born.

Henry enjoyed being groomed almost as much as he did his watermelon, and I recall going into his paddock, brushes in hand, combing out his long mane and shining up his dapples. It was a time before ShowSheen mane and tail detanglers, and the Cowboy Magic detangler of that time was once handed to me by a team roper: a can of WD-40.

I had told Henry on occasion while grooming him up that one day we would raise his stud fee and change his name to the more sophisticated French-sounding Henri, yet Henry just seemed like a Henry, and so he remained.

He was bred to mostly Thoroughbred mares, and the high-withered, stringy-necked ones often produced the best crosses.

Henry was big—weighing in at almost 2,200 pounds—and somewhat, shall we say, oversized in ways that precluded him from being able to breed the lighter Thoroughbred mares naturally. It was therefore necessary to collect him artificially using the "jump mare" I had at the clinic.

A jump mare, by the way, is not so called because "jumps" such as fences or cross rails are involved. She is called a jump mare because she is willing to get jumped on by a stallion.

Serendipity was the jump mare I used to collect Henry

off of. I had spayed her when she was a two-year-old filly, and having no ovaries meant that she wasn't capable of producing progesterone, the hormone that keeps mares out of heat. A 3 cc injection of estrogen would bring her into a standing heat within hours.

Serendipity was well suited for the job. She was a well-muscled, beefy rear-ended Appaloosa Quarter horse–type mare and was just sturdy enough to be able to support Henry's one-ton enormity. As Henry mounted her, I would deflect his erect penis off to the side into an artificial vagina, a heated and lubricated water jacket into which he would ejaculate. Using the collected semen, I would then artificially inseminate the mare that Henry was booked to breed.

It was late that California spring, and two of the mares that Henry had successfully bred had foaled and were returning to be re-bred. The mares had their foals by their sides when they arrived at the clinic.

Boxcar Willy was a not-so-little, charcoal-gray stud colt, and Tanqueray was a dark bay and still somewhat dainty filly despite being half Percheron. She eventually developed Henry's beefy musculature and her owners would simply call her Tank.

It was a week or so after both mares were inseminated and returned home that I noticed Henry walking slowly, with his giant head just barely off the ground. As I walked up to him, he didn't lift his head to greet me or sniff my pocket for a treat as he ordinarily did. I hurriedly walked back to the paddock gate, grabbed his halter, placed it over his head, and tried to pull his head up. As I slowly tried to elevate his head, he grunted and his expression became one of anxiety and pain. Again I tried, despite his objections, but was unable to raise it.

Henry's paddock was on a slow-rising hill at the top of which was an open-sided turnout shed constructed from old creosote-treated power poles. I would frequently see him rubbing his massive neck on the pole uprights that supported the shed. In fact, he enjoyed his power pole massages so much that several areas of the pressure-treated poles were polished where he rubbed. I suspected that Henry must have picked up a splinter while rubbing his neck. I had seen this before in horses that liked to rub, and it was all too easy to pick up a sliver of wood from a fence board or old barn siding.

I carefully examined Henry's neck, thinking that perhaps hidden under his mane, embedded under the skin, I would find some localized swelling or draining tract that would suggest a foreign body such as a fragment of wood. Yet there was nothing I could find that was visibly unusual or palpably different.

Over the course of two months, I tried every medication I had in the back of my truck, including muscle relaxants, anti-inflammatories, antispasmodics, powerful-acting corticosteroids, sedatives, and potent injectable analgesics. Time and rest were often sure-bet remedies for any number of injuries in horses, but they didn't help either.

Henry's neck muscles were beginning to atrophy and hollow out, suggesting the likelihood of nerve damage. Muscle tissue needs an intact nerve supply not only to function but to retain its normal symmetry and size. Yet if there was some sort of spinal nerve compression or injury in Henry's neck, how would I know where? There was no X-ray machine in any hospital powerful enough to see through the complex vertebral structural anatomy of Henry's enormous neck. It would be like trying to do an MRI on an elephant.

I was frustrated at not knowing what I could do to help, and even more so because I felt I had the background and training that should provide me with some insight as to how to do so.

June had slipped into July and it was a typical cloudless summer day in central California: dusty, dry, and hot. It was close on noon and already 110 degrees. The winter rains wouldn't arrive until October or perhaps November.

I was out vaccinating some horses at Lynn Sander's farm, a neighbor about a mile down the road, and mentioned briefly what had happened to Henry. "You should call Dave," she said. "He might be able to help." I knew that Lynn's husband, Dave, was a chiropractor in town, but as I waved good-bye and pulled out the driveway, I thought to myself, "How could a chiropractor possibly help a patient that weighed more than a ton?"

Time was passing and nothing changed. Henry was depressed, losing weight and in pain. I felt helpless and grappled with what I sensed needed to be done. He certainly wasn't enjoying any kind of quality life and I was becoming guilty of what I so frequently criticized my horse clients for: not having the courage to do the right thing. As sad as it was, it was unfair to Henry to keep him going. It would break my heart to have to put him down and yet there seemed little else to do.

I was driving past Lynn's house that afternoon and thought about her suggestion. The word "chiropractic" was hardly mentioned in any courses I had in veterinary school, and chiropractic certainly couldn't be taken seriously as being therapeutic in the world of equine veterinary medicine. My veterinary professors in orthopedic surgery seemed more than cynical when questions about chiropractic medicine were raised. It was considered "alternative," "clinically irrelevant," and besides, chiropractors weren't real doctors.

It was a last resort but somehow, later that day, I found myself calling information from my cell phone and asking for Dave's office. "Doctor Sander's office. May I help you?" the receptionist asked. I paused for a moment before saying anything, wondering what I was doing. "Hello, this is Doctor Sander's office. May I help you?" she asked again.

"Uh, yes, I'm a neighbor of Dave's and I was wondering if I could speak with him for a moment," I replied.

"He's with a patient right now. Can the doctor give you a call back?"

It was the following day, and as the car pulled up to the clinic, I called out, "Hey, Dave, good to see you." As we walked over to Henry's paddock together, I explained what little I knew about what had happened. "He's been like this for two months, losing weight, depressed and in pain. I'm not sure what you can do for him . . . I've already tried everything."

These last few words slipped out before I knew I had said them. I didn't want Dave to think my calling him was an act of desperation, a drums-and-chicken-feathers sort of move on my part, even though of course I knew that it was. Dave was kind enough to pretend he didn't hear the remark and we arrived outside Henry's paddock.

Henry stood quietly with his head hanging as Dave methodically began to slowly and deliberately palpate his thick neck. There was a "Humph," an "Interesting," which was followed by a "Hmmm . . . ," and then a "That's odd," a "Sure is tight," and then a "Yup! That's it."

"What's it?" I asked "Whadda ya mean, that's it?"

Dave didn't answer but looked around the clinic and,

glancing at the grassy lawn area behind the barn, asked, "Can you knock him out for me?"

"You mean give him a general anesthetic?" I replied. "Yeah, sure I can do that. I can lay him out for thirty minutes or so. Is that enough time? So what did you find, Dave?"

"He's subluxated his C6 cervical vertebra resulting in compression of one of the pair of spinal nerves," he responded. "The C6 impairment at the root of the spinal nerve is resulting in pain and paralysis," he added.

"You mean you think he's got a pinched nerve?" I asked.

"I know so," he confidently responded.

"Can you help him?" I asked.

"Yup, but in order to correct the subluxation, I'll need him completely out," Dave explained.

"I'll be right back with what we need," I said, heading toward my truck.

I smirked and shook my head, however, as I grabbed a couple of vials and some syringes from one of the cabinets in my truck. "Radiculopathy" happens to be the fancy medical term for a compressed spinal nerve root or radicle as it comes out of the vertebra and how appropriately "ridiculous" I thought to myself was Dave's presumptuous C6 diagnosis.

We led Henry over to a large, grassy, round pen behind the clinic where I would lay horses down for any number of short-term surgical procedures. The ground was grass covered, soft, and being a round pen, there were no corners to get injured on when the horses came out of the anesthesia.

I gave Henry an IV triple cocktail of Rompun, Valium, and Torb in his jugular vein. As big and heavy as the draft breeds are, they're actually lightweights when it comes to sedatives and anesthetics. Within less than a minute Henry was swaying back and forth and ready for the ketamine to follow, which would drop him.

"Can you get him right side up?" Dave shouted from outside the pen. I wondered if Dave had any idea what he was asking. I was holding on to the lead rope of 2,000-plus pounds of horse which was about to topple in a heap, and Dave wanted him right side up.

As Henry started to buckle, I heaved his head to the right so he would fall on his left side. It worked. I placed a towel over his eyes and looked at Dave, feeling slightly miffed, and said, "Right side up. He'll be out for half an hour or so. Do what you think you can do."

Dave came over to this Goliath of a horse lying unconscious on the ground and placed both of his knees on Henry's neck. In a circular motion, using his knees over Henry's mid-cervical vertebral column, he was "manipulating" Henry. Dave explained that because of Henry's size he wasn't able to perform the manipulation with his hands but could do it with his knees.

"That sounds like a bit of a stretch," I said, saying what I was thinking before I had a chance to take it back. "Um, what I meant was: Do you think that's something you can really do?" I asked.

Dave was focused and continued to slowly rotate his knees over the midportion of Henry's neck.

It was just about half an hour later when Henry started to come out of the anesthesia, and another few minutes before he stood up, a bit wobbly and his head still down. After leading him slowly back to his paddock, I returned to the barn to chat with Dave for twenty minutes or so and wait for the anesthesia to completely wear off.

"It's time, let's go have a look," I said to Dave.

We began to head out the barn toward Henry's paddock

when all of a sudden I remembered I had forgotten something. “Oh, wait just a sec, Dave, I’ll be right back,” I said. I dashed back into the barn office and opened the door to the fridge. It was my private stash in the salad drawer: several slices of watermelon.

“What’d you forget?” Dave asked when I met him outside the barn and we headed over to Henry’s paddock.

“Ah, it’s kind of silly but the big guy likes watermelon,” I said, showing him the slice of melon I had in my hand.

Henry was standing quietly in the middle of his paddock with his head still hanging down when Dave and I opened up the gate and walked in. “C’mon Henry, look what I’ve got, big guy,” I said in a loud voice, holding up the piece of melon for him to see.

His response would normally have been to lift his head and come trotting down his paddock hill for his watermelon treat. Overshadowed by pain and paralysis, however, it seemed that such a simple pleasure would no longer be. I felt both sad and discouraged as I lowered my raised hand holding the slice of watermelon. “Thanks for trying,” I said to Dave.

We headed out the paddock gates, and it was then that we heard the hoofbeats. We turned around to see Henry trotting our way with his head held high.

Henry stopped in front of us expectantly. I smiled to see him munch on the juicy rind of melon, his eyes glassy and trancelike, the watermelon juice running down his chin.

I thanked Dave over and over as we walked back to his car, and when I tried to pay him, he wouldn’t let me. As he got in his car and turned the ignition on, I reached through the window, shook his hand, thanked him again, and said, “Great job, Doc.”

{SEVEN}

A Jewel of a Mom

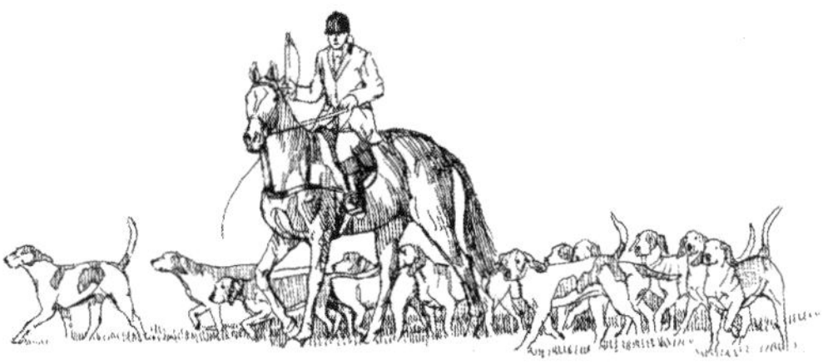

"AYE, SHE'S GOT A BIT OF A GIMP but she's not really lame," is perhaps how an Irish horse trader would have described my Thoroughbred mare Jewel. Of course, any horse with a bit of a gimp is in fact lame, the exception being the one the Irish horse trader is trying to sell you.

Jewel was indeed a bit lame. She had three titanium screws in her right front ankle from a fracture that left her with a head bob, not so obvious at a walk, but more so at a trot.

Jewel was a ten-year-old, stringy-necked, dark bay Thoroughbred mare given to me by the local foxhunt in Santa Ynez, California. She was retired now, no longer able to do what she once loved to do. She had raced on the track prior to coming to the hunt, and although she wasn't fast enough for the track, she was plenty quick enough to be a good mount for a "whipper-in." She was nimble, clever, and caught on quickly to the job she came to look forward to as a hunt horse. She had the necessary agility and speed that a whipper-in's horse needed to give chase to the swift coyote that made their home in the central coast mountains of California.

Our foxhunt was fortunate to have the opportunity to hunt on several large cattle ranches along the coastal foothills. The ranchers knew we appreciated the chance to foxhunt on their land, and we in turn were careful not to disturb the cows when we came across them milling about at the watering holes or grazing along the hillsides.

It was an early morning in mid-November and we were hunting on the Jack Ranch, an enormous cattle ranch nestled in the foothills north of Santa Barbara. The winter rains, which would transform the golden-brown hills to lush and fertile grazing grounds, had yet to arrive. The grass-covered hillsides were still brown and dry from the hot summer and the parched ground hard after eight months or more without rain. In the hollows of the canyons, the Spanish moss hung eerily from the oak trees where a fog had moved in from the coast during the night. The crisp morning air heightened the wonderful earthy smells of the low-lying sagebrush and the cattle that had passed through during the night.

The field was scarcely mounted—a few riders had just managed to put a toe in the stirrup iron while others had barely passed a flask back to its owner—when one of the masters up ahead looked back and motioned to quiet the chat. The hounds had been cast and seemed unusually eager. They soon gave full cry to the fresh scent of coyote. We were off!

The field galloped on to try and keep up, but the huntsman, whips, and the hounds moved quickly out of sight.

The sloped terrain with many a ditch and bank allowed only the most fit and agile of horses and riders to keep up with the hounds.

The field was making its way at a trot down the side of a scrubby sagebrush-covered hill when we saw in the clearing ahead one of the whips off his horse. He was kneeling to the side, running his hands down one of the horse's front legs. I asked the master to be excused from the field, trotted over, and dismounted to have a closer look.

"What happened?" I asked, as I felt the mare's right front ankle, now almost twice the size of her left front. Perplexed and clearly distracted by the mare's sudden injury, the rider tried to recall what had happened. "We were right behind the hounds when we jumped across that dry river bed. She took two funny strides and I pulled her up."

"It's a good thing you did," I said, as I felt the crepitus behind her ankle. "Feel this." I placed his hand behind her fetlock. "Now, gently press. It feels sort of like you're crunching Rice Krispies, the way it kind of crinkles and crackles. I'm pretty sure she's fractured her ankle, but I think the cannon bone is okay."

I stayed alone with Jewel as the whip headed off on my horse back to the trailers. The swelling in her ankle was from blood and the crepitus or crackling I felt was the grating of bone fragments.

I stroked her neck and calmed her with my voice. She had a worried eye. She knew it was serious and being the intelligent Thoroughbred that she was, she stood still, somehow knowing that to try and move would only make matters worse. She was intuitively correct, for if she had tried to take a weight-bearing step on her fractured limb, she indeed would have made matters much worse.

Bone fractures in horses and humans alike are of two kinds. In a "closed" fracture the skin is intact over the break in the limb. A "compound" or "open" fracture is one where the fracture has torn through the overlying skin. Attempting to bear weight on what initially is a closed fracture can result in the sharp-ended fracture fragments tearing the overlying skin, resulting in an open fracture.

Horses arriving at a surgical referral hospital with a closed fracture have a much more favorable prognosis of survival than horses with an open fracture. The bacterial contamination which invariably occurs in an open fracture is why. The osteomyelitis —or bone infection—in an open fracture is a complication that drastically alters the prognosis from favorable to one suggesting where the horse will most likely end up: grave.

I kept all sorts of emergency gear in the gooseneck of the horse trailer, including plenty of bandages, cotton, and medications. However, PVC pipe splints and clamps for stabilizing a leg fracture for transport were items I kept back at the clinic. We would have to improvise a splint.

I heard the whipper-in driving back with my trailer rattling down the dirt road between the canyons. Jewel would have to walk a quarter mile or more before we would be able to reach the road.

"Stay with her, keep her quiet, and don't let her move. I'll be back in half an hour," I instructed the whipper-in when he returned. I handed him the reins and calmly walked a few steps in the direction of the trailer, disappeared behind some scrub brush, and then began to run.

Out of breath, I flung the tack room door of the trailer open and scrambled to find all the tape, bandaging, cotton, and polo wraps I could find. What could I use to splint her leg? I thought frantically as I looked around the tack room. I glanced at the broom and the manure fork. *Got it!* I could break off the handles of the broom and the manure fork and use them to splint and stabilize the fracture. I took the broom outside and set one end on the tire of the truck, the other end on the ground, and jumped. The handle snapped in two. I did the same with the manure fork, then broke off the sharp-ended pieces as best I could and headed back.

"How's she doing?" I asked the whipper-in.

"She's been quiet. She hasn't tried to take a step," he replied.

"Good. Keep hanging on to her. Love on her a little bit, stroke her neck, talk to her, and tell her she's brave. This is going to take a few minutes," I said.

I knelt down by Jewel's right front leg and began to tape and wrap her leg, incorporating the broken wooden handles of the broom and manure fork as tightly as I could to minimize any movement of the fracture site that might occur on the walk back to the trailer.

Although it would take almost an hour for Jewel to hobble back to the trailer, we made it. "Hang on just a minute," I said to the whipper-in before we loaded her up. "Let me tape and tighten her splint a bit more."

Transporting a horse with a broken leg in a trailer has the potential to make matters worse. The jostling about in a trailer can easily destabilize and displace the fracture fragments further. A closed fracture can become an open fracture and instead of the one or two fracture fragments before the horse got onto the trailer, there are now four or five. It happens all too frequently that a horse with a broken leg has a fair prognosis of survival until it is put on a trailer to be shipped to the surgical referral facility.

"What do you think?" the whipper-in asked as I knelt down by Jewel's leg, reinforcing the splint with tourniquet-like wraps of even more tape to ensure the stability of the fracture site.

"This is a career-ender. She'll never be able to hunt again," I responded.

Jewel was a brave mare, I thought to myself as she hobbled up the ramp of the trailer and let me squeeze her in between the two slanted panel gates inside. She could lean and brace against them to catch her balance for the two-hour-long trip to the referral hospital.

The surgeons at the referral clinic met us as we pulled in. I had called ahead to let them know what had happened and that we were on the way. They managed to properly stabilize the leg before taking Jewel off the trailer and into the hospital for X-rays. The radiographs revealed a fractured proximal sesamoid bone in her ankle. It would require an expensive surgery to repair the fracture, the outcome of which would result in Jewel being pasture-sound at best, a lawn ornament of sorts, never to be ridden again.

Based on finances alone, the decision to spend several thousand dollars to repair the broken leg of a not-so-successful Thoroughbred racehorse is questionable at best. The surgery would be a salvage procedure. Jewel's prospects as a broodmare would be another losing proposition. Breeding a mare that had never stood in the winner's circle in hopes of getting future racehorse winners would be a long shot and financially foolish.

Jewel was owned by the master of the hunt, who was a businessman. His family had a big name in tires and other interests, including their own California wine label. He was also a compassionate man and elected to go ahead with the costly surgery and rehabilitation involved in repairing the fracture in Jewel's ankle. The surgery would essentially involve a few titanium screws, a cast, and several months of rest.

The winter rains had come to the central coast of California, and it was in the spring that I saw Jewel again. I had received a phone call with a very generous offer from the master of the hunt. He knew I had a Percheron draft horse stallion and wondered if I would be interested in being given Jewel as a broodmare. He felt that it would be a shame to retire her at such a young age and that perhaps she could find a new career as a broodmare to produce future foxhunters. His gift to me of Jewel also came with the offer that the hunt would buy back all her foals.

The first of Jewel's foals by my Percheron draft horse stallion, Henry, was a beefy little colt that quickly grew into his name of Amtrak. It was Jewel's second foal, however, that won my heart. She was a little filly, and inherited from Jewel the refined, delicate, and intelligent attributes of the Thoroughbred. From Henry, she inherited wonderfully big feet and a quiet spirit.

She was born on the dainty and frail side of life, however, despite her drafty sire. Around the third day after she was born, I began to sense that something wasn't right. Initially she just seemed not as playful and curious about life as one would expect a foal to be. It was a day or so later, however, I noticed that she was grinding her teeth, drooling ropey strands of saliva, and lying upside down in her stall, all of the typical clinical signs of a foal with gastric ulcers.

A lot of Thoroughbred foals are born with stress ulcers. It seems that in the quest to breed a faster horse, other desirable genetic traits have inadvertently been edged off the Thoroughbred chromosome. Clearly, the Ferrari can't also be the Land Rover, and perhaps "sturdy," "robust," and "hardy" are being bred out as speed is encrypted in.

Zantac is the trade name for ranitidine, an anti-ulcer medication used for people and horses alike. I started the filly on several pills three times a day. The medication would raise the pH of her stomach toward a more alkaline and less acidic state. I also treated her with a medication called Carafate, which goes to work as an "ulcer putty" in the stomach. It's an orally administered spackling compound of sorts, used to fill in and coat the erosive pitting in the gastric lining.

Coffee grinders are a huge time-saver in equine clinics. Rather than try to mortar and pestle pills needed to medicate the foal, I would count out her pill dose of Zantac and Carafate tablets, place them in the coffee grinder, and presto. Using a 60 cc dose syringe, I would then mix her powdered pills with a couple of ounces of liquid strawberry yogurt.

Although initially a bit hesitant about being caught up and restrained to be given her medicine, she quickly realized how good it actually tasted. Most foals quickly acquire a taste for liquid strawberry yogurt, and she was no exception. Within less than twenty-four hours of having started on her anti-ulcer medication, she was not only acting more like a normal foal, but would daintily trot over when I opened the stall door, eagerly anticipating what was about to happen.

I would gently cradle her head and neck while slipping the syringe into her mouth. As I slowly pushed the plunger of the syringe, the sound of eager slurps would follow. It was then that I would smile while watching her close her eyes in obvious delight.

Every few weeks I would try to discontinue the medication, in hopes that her gastric ulcers had healed, only to find that the depression, salivating, and teeth-grinding would return. I would wait to name her, I thought, until I knew she was going to be well.

It would be six months before her gastric ulcers had healed and I was able to discontinue the medication.

On a cool summer morning, as I walked down to the barn, I watched the filly in her paddock running, bucking, and clearly feeling as if she could grab the clouds out of the sky. *Hmmm . . . ,* I thought to myself, *I wonder what would be a good name for her?* Something easy to say, I thought, and perhaps a name that might rhyme with that of her brother Amtrak.

Amtrak and his sister Zantac would eventually take up the same career that their mother, Jewel, had so enjoyed, as hunt horses in the coastal hills of California.

{EIGHT}

The Young Man and the Sea

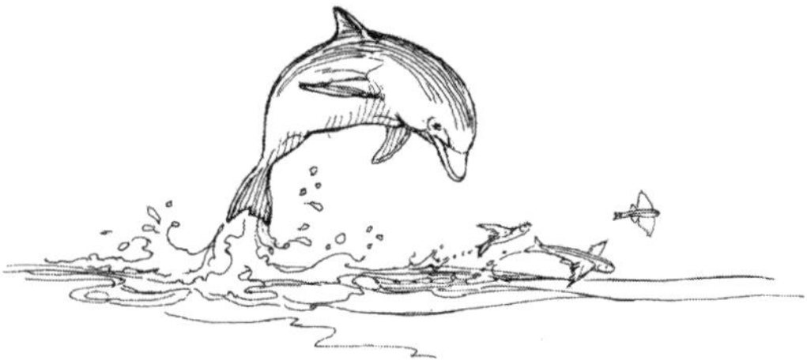

I STOOD ON THE DECK OF THE FREIGHTER SS *Austral Endurance*, looking back at the giant dockside cranes that had just stacked and loaded the last of the containers onto the deck of the ship. It was two o'clock in the morning and we were finally under way, leaving the harbor at Port Elizabeth, New Jersey. I was headed for Australia to work on a sheep and cattle ranch.

It was July and I had just turned eighteen. It felt good to be leaving my life in New York despite not really knowing where I was going. I was at sea but also very much adrift. At sea and lost, or I suppose just lost at sea, it didn't matter. My life seemed without direction or purpose.

The journey that most of my classmates had embarked upon from boarding school seemed to be one chosen by others. The direct path of college and a career in banking, business, or law was a choice that didn't seem to be entirely theirs but rather one that was swayed by tradition and parental prodding. Nonetheless, of the two roads that diverged in the wood, theirs at least seemed to be enviably safe, secure, and promising.

Wayward and yet adventurous would be the next few years of my life. It wasn't really a conscious realization but in many ways my journey would be about finding my dad in my life. I missed him and hadn't seen him in ten years and wouldn't for several years more. Even then we would have only a few days.

The *Austral Endurance* was a type of freighter called a container vessel. In contrast to a tanker that ships crude oil or a traditional bulk cargo vessel that ships grain or coal, container vessels carry their entire load in truck-size containers.

The big-rig semi trucks you see on the highways are often hauling these containers to and from shipping ports.

The *Austral Endurance* was a midsize freighter with a capacity of about eight hundred containers. The ship's crew consisted of the captain, three mates, a chief engineer, three assistant engineers, several "oilers" whose jobs involved doing what their name implies, and a kitchen crew of three. There were also six passengers, of which I was one.

After we had sailed south for several days in the Atlantic Ocean, the color of the water became an indigo blue, the clouds more cumulus, and the air more humid. We were in the tropics of the Caribbean Sea, sailing toward Central America.

The sea voyage would last almost a month and I would spend seemingly countless hours during the day at the bow of the ship. The waves from the bow of the ship were a ready source of amusement and merriment for the occasional pod of dolphins, and the fact that flying fish are on the dolphin's menu would make for quite an entertaining show.

Dolphins leapt playfully through the waves thrown up by the ship, making surrounding schools of flying fish think they were the target of a predatory chase. Of course, the escape tactic of a flying fish is to flee by flying and that's precisely what they would do. The "wings" of the fish are actually its pectoral fins, and a "flight" is really more of a 45 mph glide of about 150 feet. As the dolphins leapt in and out of the waves, the synchronous response of hundreds of flying fish would be to take flight across the bow of the ship.

If I wasn't on deck staring off in wonder at the ocean expanse, I was chatting with the crew about their life at sea. They appreciated my curiosity about their lives on board a freighter and in turn allowed me to spend time with them as they worked on the bridge or down below deck with the oilers in the engine room.

I had brought books by the great Russian novelists that everyone is supposed to read, but there wasn't enough time. *War and Peace*, *Anna Karenina*, and *The Brothers Karamazov* would have to wait. I was dreamy and content to lie on the deck at night, smelling the warm salt breeze and watching for hours the dozens of shooting stars.

THE REALIZATION WAS STRANGE. What cost thirty thousand people their lives and took ten years to construct was but a day's travel through a series of steps made of water. The fifty-mile Panama Canal raises and lowers ships hundreds of feet through a series of locks as they sail between the Atlantic and the Pacific. Sadly, at the time when the Panama Canal was under construction in 1904, little was understood about the role of the mosquito in the transmission of yellow fever and malaria, diseases that would take the lives of so many workers.

After two weeks of calm seas in the Pacific, a day's voyage remained to reach Sydney. The Pacific Ocean is for the most part aptly named except for a stretch between New Zealand and Australia known as the Tasman Sea, where the waters can be tempestuous.

I was informed by the ship's crew that it would be best not to go on deck that day, but of course, being the age that I was, adventure and excitement took precedence over safety. Feeling somewhat like a stowaway, I was careful not to be seen as I made my way up to the bow of the ship and waited as we sailed toward the storm. Oh, I'm sure it wasn't a real tropical storm with thirty-foot waves and cyclone winds and such, but I was young and it seemed so to me.

From the bow of the ship I could see the dark and foreboding clouds off in the distance. As the winds gusted and the sea began to surge and swell, the big ship would slowly heave in rhythm with the waves.

I was crouched between the on-deck steel containers, watching in awe as the storm waves began to break over the bow of the freighter and slam into the containers around me. Safeguarded and shielded between the steel containers from the impact of the waves, I could hear the holding cables that lashed the on-deck containers strain and creak.

Drenched in sea spray, alone amidst the sounds of the waves breaking over the bow and against the containers around me, I was exhilarated. It mattered little that the afternoon hours would pass well into the darkness of night before I could venture out from my place of safety and hiding. I convinced myself that I dare not move until the storm passed as I would surely have been swept overboard in a moment by one of the powerful waves had I tried to make my way back along the deck.

I'm sure there was a bit of imaginary development as to the perils of the late afternoon and evening and yet, if ever there had been a *Sea Wolf* comic book, I was certainly lost in the fantasy of its pages.

My absence at the galley dinner table that evening would be of little concern to the kitchen crew and would likely draw a few chuckles. The oilers and engineers would probably attribute my empty chair to a young landlubber's bout of seasickness from what they would perceive as a mere bit of rough sailing.

The freighter docked in Sydney the following day, and in less than a week I was mustering sheep in the outback of Western Australia.

{NINE}

Toke of the Town

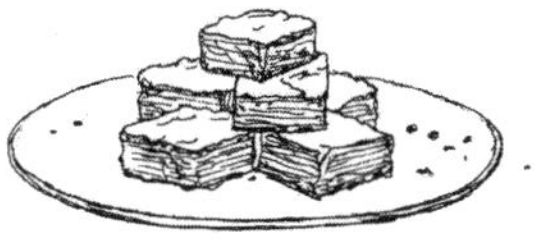

"WANT A HIT? IT'S PRETTY GOOD WEED," Miles asked me.

"No, thanks. I'm good," I responded, rolling down the passenger side window of his vet truck.

I was in Mendocino, California, and the Grateful Dead's "Truckin" was what we were listening to as we drove north on Highway 1. It was a beautiful blue-sky day in July. The Pacific Ocean was on our left and a magnificent stretch of California redwood forest was on our right.

Mendocino is an old logging town in northern California that sits on a coastal bluff overlooking the Pacific Ocean. It's a favored and languorous place for artists, poets, and seals alike.

Hundreds of chocolate-brown, bulbous bodies often laze on the rocky promontories that jut out into the sea below the small town of Mendocino. Their lives are enviable as they bask in the sun in a part of the world where the sea has a gentle sweep, the water is calm, and the going is easy. Hours can slip by watching the seal pups bobbing playfully in the water or their parents having a pleasant roll in the sand.

Mendocino is also part of the Redwood Coast, where two-thousand-year-old redwood trees grow taller than the Statue of Liberty. Rugged cliffs, rocky tide pools, sandy beaches, and redwood forests make it a pretty magical part of the world. Seal Rock is just that, and Pelican Bay is a place where you can watch brown pelicans plunge for fish. If you use a pair of binoculars you can see the fish in the pelican's throat pouch, fighting the good fight before it is swallowed.

Mendocino is also where my classmate Miles from veterinary school had his horse practice.

After completing our residency programs together at the veterinary school in Davis, California, we set up our own equine practices in different parts of the state. Miles moved north to Mendocino, a place of both remarkable beauty and everything alternative.

I had always wanted to see Mendocino, so when Miles asked me to come spend a few days with him, the decision was easy. I rescheduled some appointments and headed north.

Miles grew up in the hustle and bustle of LA and wanted out. He had worked as a kid with a track vet at the Santa Anita Park and loved working with the horses but didn't care for the racehorse industry. He was plenty bright, wanted to spend his life working with horses, and was interested not so much in making money as in a change of lifestyle.

Amidst several equine veterinary journals on the seat of his vet truck was a recent issue of *Toke of the Town*, a news publication about everything cannabis. "Think green" to

Miles was a California concept that was less about recycling and more about the legalization of marijuana. He had been a Grateful Dead jam band fan ever since we met and evidently not much had changed since I had seen him last.

"So where we headed?" I asked as Miles took another hit.

"We got a lameness exam to do on a dressage horse. You mind if I turn this next one up. They did this one live," Miles said, turning up the volume on "Going Down the Road Feeling Bad".

"Here we are," Miles said, turning down a driveway between several redwoods. "Kelley's got some nice-moving high-dollar dressage horses. Not sure what the problem is but we'll figure it out when we get there."

"Wow . . . this is some place," I said to Miles as we drove into a near magical clearing in the midst of a forest.

"Yeah, she and Billy did it up right," Miles responded. We pulled up in front of the barn and got out of the truck, but Miles kept the music going, wanting to hear the last of the song. Kelley came out of the barn. "Sounds familiar," she said, smiling. "I've heard that one before."

Miles introduced me to Kelley as we headed into the barn where a horse was standing on the cross ties, tacked up. "He's a beauty. What's his breed?" I asked.

"Thanks, his name is Rousseau and he's an eight-year-old Dutch," Kelley replied.

The Netherlands are famous for producing some of the world's most talented dressage and jumping horses. The Dutch warmblood as a dressage horse is essentially a 1,400-pound ballet dancer—fluid, elegant, and graceful. As a jumper, the breed is bold, forward, powerful, and capable of effortlessly jumping a five-foot-wide oxer. News of a Dutch horse bringing home gold or silver in the Olympics in either dressage or jumping isn't quite ho-hum but almost.

"So tell me what's been going on," Miles asked Kelley.

"I'm not sure, but something's not right. There's nothing obvious that I can see when I lunge him and nothing I can consistently feel that's off when I'm riding him, but I know he's not right," Kelley replied. "He's talented tons as an upper-level Prix St. Georges horse, and perhaps I've been pushing him a bit more than I should have. I just don't know."

"Do you sense he's not right in a particular gait, or is it more to the left or right?" Miles asked.

"It's not so much a gait or a direction but more the lateral work that seems to be difficult for him," she responded.

"Let's take him out to the dressage ring and have you ride him," Miles said to Kelley. "We'll meet you out there" he added, and Miles and I headed out the back of the barn toward the ring.

"What would you like us to do?" Kelley asked. "Warm him up a bit and then we'll put him to work," Miles replied.

"I can't see anything yet," I said to Miles as we watched Kelley warm up Rousseau at the walk and trot from the side of the ring. Miles didn't respond but remained focused on Rousseau.

"All right, Kelley, have him trot to the left on a twenty-meter circle and then to the right," Miles said. "Okay, that's good. Now some canter circles to the left and right," Miles instructed.

Lameness exams on horses are much more diagnostic if the horse is being ridden in a circle rather than in a straight line. The weight placed on the inside fore and hind limb is greater, and a lameness that is difficult to see on a straight line becomes more evident.

"Okay, Kelley, he's warmed up enough. Let's start to collect him up and see what we've got," Miles said.

Miles had Kelley do some lateral work, including some leg yields, shoulder-ins and half passes in an attempt to appreciate any subtle change of gait or rhythm.

"How's the contact on the bit, Kelley? Does it seem heavier in one direction than the other?" Miles asked. "Now ride him on the wrong diagonal," he instructed Kelley.

Ordinarily, as the horse is ridden to the left or right on a circle, the rider posts out of the saddle when the inside limb is weight bearing. Riding on the "wrong diagonal" means that the rider is sitting when they should be rising out of the saddle, which has the effect of altering the balance of the horse.

Subtle lamenesses are just that: they are elusive and difficult to detect. Attempts to deliberately shift the horse off balance even slightly may be of investigative value in diagnosing an obscure lameness.

"Something is not quite right," Miles commented. "See how he's not tracking up in his left hind and he hesitates when asked for a lead change to the right at the canter. The rhythm of the stride and swing isn't there. He seems resistant, not engaged, and doesn't have the freedom in his back to get round, come up, and collect."

Miles performed several flexion tests, had Kelley longe Rousseau at the trot and canter without her riding him, and methodically palpated the long muscles of the horse's back and croup. He then palpated the flexor tendons and suspensory ligaments of Rousseau's hind limbs and found him to be a bit "flinchy" high in his left rear suspensory ligament.

"Let's take him back to the barn, take the tack off, and

put him on the cross ties. We'll grab some gear from the truck and meet you back inside."

"What do you think?" I asked Miles as we walked back toward his vet truck.

"He's back sore, can't engage, and I bet if we scan his left hind we'll find something," Miles replied.

Miles returned to the barn with his ultrasound machine. He explained to Kelley that Rousseau had lower back pain, which was likely secondary to a left rear limb lameness.

"It's not that he *can't* collect and engage, it's just painful when he does," Miles explained to Kelley as he applied some ultrasound gel to Rousseau's left hind leg. "I'm pretty sure that he has an inflamed suspensory ligament and he's using his back muscles to compensate for what is painful to do with his left hind."

Miles sounded a bit like a chapter out of a diagnostic ultrasound book as he described out loud the changes he saw on the ultrasound screen while he scanned Rousseau's hind limb. "Do you see this? Here's an area of echolucency in the proximal suspensory that makes it difficult to marginate the borders of the medial aspect of the ligament. The suspensory doesn't appear as uniform and homogeneous as it should, which indicates the likelihood of blood and edema within the ligament."

"What's all that mean? Is he going to be okay?" Kelley asked.

"He has a slight tear in his suspensory but good news is, we caught it early," Miles explained. "It's a good thing you didn't just bute him up and try and push him through it. That would have just made the injury worse.

"It's painful for him to extend and reach with his left hind, so he's trying to use the long muscles of his back to compensate. He's back sore, can't collect and engage because he's lame in his left rear."

Miles explained to Kelley that tendons and ligaments are slow to heal because of their poor blood supply, and outlined a therapeutic plan for Rousseau that would require a layup period of several months. "He'll be okay but it's gonna take time and work on your part to bring him back sound. He'll need to be on a little low-dose bute to help cut the pain and swelling, and you'll have to take him out of work, put him on a limited exercise program, and ice the leg three to four times a day for the first couple of weeks. After that you'll be sweating the leg with some DMSO, and I'll need to scan him every month or so to make sure he's on the mend."

"Of course, I'll do whatever needs to be done. Do you think that this is my fault, I mean maybe I was working him too hard and asking for too much?" Kelley wanted to know.

"Life's big paradox is horses," Miles responded. "They look big and powerful but they break easy."

Miles was meticulous in writing out a detailed treatment plan for Kelley to follow to rehab Rousseau from his suspensory ligament injury. Kelley was of course relieved to know that Rousseau would be sound in a few months, able to go back to work, and fortunately, she had other horses to ride while Rousseau was laid up.

"I made some brownies earlier. C'mon up to the kitchen and have some before you guys go," Kelley said as we packed up our gear in the back of the vet truck.

"Sure thing," Miles answered.

"I'll meet you guys up at the house. Head over when you're ready," Kelley said.

Kelley's house was elaborately designed and constructed

as nothing short of a spectacular redwood tree house. The kitchen was upstairs, and in the middle of it grew an eight-hundred-year-old, fifteen-story–tall, giant redwood. Through skylights I could see other towering redwoods and from the decking I could hear the sounds of birds and see beautiful gardens and a river.

Kelley made us each a mug of herbal tea as we chatted about Rousseau and her other horses.

"Here, have one," Kelley said to Miles, passing him a plate of brownies. "I made them just the way you like them."

"Thanks," Miles said, taking one and passing the plate to me. "Where's Billy?" he asked Kelley.

"He's in San Francisco finishing up an album, and then they have a bit of a break before going on tour."

As I took a bite of the brownie, I bit down on some seeds. *Perhaps I should have known*, I thought to myself as I put the brownie down on the napkin in front of me.

"Good to see you, Kelley. Let me know how Rousseau is doing in a couple of weeks and say hi to Billy when he gets back," Miles said.

"You want one more for the road?" Kelley asked Miles, offering him another brownie.

"Sure thing," Miles replied.

"Nice to have met you, Kelley," I said, thanking her, and Miles and I headed downstairs, out the house, and back to his vet truck.

"They did this one live too," Miles said, turning up "Dancing in the Streets" as we drove out past the redwoods, with the Pacific Ocean in view. "Check it out, here comes Billy's drum solo," Miles added.

{TEN}

Jack Daniel's for Jeremiah

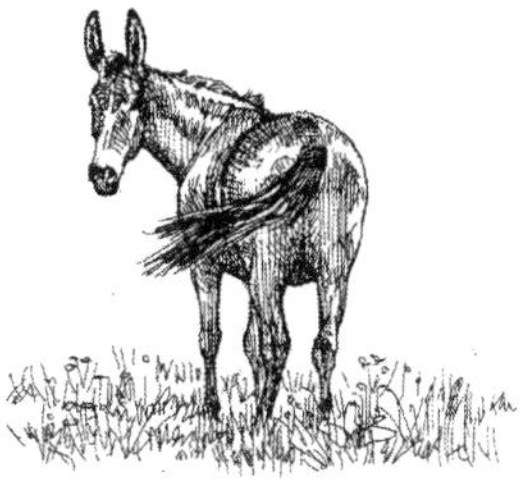

"HEY, DOC, IT'S MY JACK JEREMIAH. He's bellyachin' pretty good. I gave him a pint of bourbon and a couple shots of turpentine an' even put some brake fluid in his ears, but it ain't helped none. I'm thinkin' you better get here quick."

Clifford was a mule breeder, and mules are big business in California. Things got around in the West years ago pretty much by pack mule. They were big in prospecting, farming, freight, and mining. To this day the US Forest Service depends on mule trains to haul gear into the remote wilderness areas of national parks as well as to provide firefighters with food and supplies where helicopters and vehicles can't go.

Where my dad grew up in the Buttermilks east of the Sierra Nevada, a world-class six-day international event takes place every year. The annual Bishop Mule Days is where more than seven hundred mules compete in almost two hundred events such as calf roping, carriage driving, flat racing, and dressage. It's also a place of optimistic chatter that the likelihood of a mule bringing home the Olympic gold in dressage or show jumping is perhaps not as remote as most perceive it to be.

I turned down a dirt road and saw the sign up ahead—BRAY TELL ME FARM—pulled into the driveway, and parked outside the barn.

"Hey, Clifford, how's he doin'?" I asked, hopping out of my truck.

"It's Jeremiah and he's bellyachin' good," Clifford replied.

"I'll meet you in the barn. Let me just quickly round up some medicine," I said, and grabbed a couple of vials of sedation, some syringes, needles, and my stethoscope.

"How long has he been colicky?" I asked as I walked into the stall to find Jeremiah lying on his side.

"He's been pawin' up a storm and wantin' to roll for the last couple hours, I reckon," Clifford answered.

"Let's get him up and I'll give him a couple of injections," I said, drawing up some medication into a syringe. "Okay, Clifford, steady his head and let me get this needle into his jugular vein. This will cut the pain and relax him pretty quick." I slipped the needle into Jeremiah's vein, attached the syringe, and pushed.

"I done give him a pint of Jack Daniel's and a couple shots of turpentine but it ain't helped none," Clifford told me again. "I figured you best put a sleeve on, 'palpitate' and oil him."

"Let me have a listen on him," I said to Clifford. I passed my stethoscope over Jeremiah's chest and belly to listen to his heart rate and check to see if he had any gut sounds. "Sounds all right, Clifford. Good gut sounds and his heart rate is close on normal, so it's not the type of colic that will require belly surgery."

"That injection kicked in right quick. He's hanging his head some now," Clifford commented.

"Good, that sedation should keep him comfortable a bit longer. Let me get a sleeve from the truck, my stomach tube, and some mineral oil and I'll be right back," I said, and headed out the stall.

Jeremiah was a large, big-eared donkey and what mule breeders call a mammoth jack. He was one of two donkey sires Clifford used in his breeding program. Gus was the other, and both of them produced a lot of talented mules in the area, some of which went on to compete at Bishop and one I was told even went on to Hollywood, when Disney made a movie called *Gus*. Everybody knows that a mule can give a pretty good kick, and Disney figured to make a comedy about a mule who was a football team's star place kicker. I had been told that it was Clifford's jack that sired the mule that starred in the film.

"Hang on to him, Clifford, here we go," I said, as I squirted some lube on the shoulder-length sleeve I had just slipped on.

"He's still looking pretty out of it from that injection you give him. He ain't gonna try an' kick, Doc, you can 'palpitate' him," Clifford said.

Horse owners like to sound somewhat knowledgeable about veterinary procedures when it comes to their animals. The timing, however, just never seemed quite right for me to correct them while examining their colicky horse that "palpitating" is something one's heart does and "palpating" is something one's hand does.

Jeremiah's big ears came up as I pulled his tail to the

side and slid my arm up beyond my elbow into his rectum.

"Can you feel what's wrong with him?" Clifford asked.

I advanced my arm a bit further. "Hang on a sec, something feels kind of strange," I said. Ordinarily, manure is what a veterinarian first encounters when a rectal palpation is performed. I was feeling something entirely different, however. It felt like there was something moving, in fact many things moving. I withdrew my arm from Jeremiah's rectum to find my sleeve covered with hundreds of four- to six-inch-long cylindrically shaped worms.

"Have a look, Clifford," I said, showing him the spaghetti-like covering on my sleeve. "He's colicking because he's impacted, plugged up with a ball of roundworms," I explained.

"I can't believe it. I've been giving him tobacco juice every couple months since I got him. It's what we always did on the farm back in Tennessee for worms," Clifford exclaimed.

"I'll give you some dewormer to give him tomorrow, but right now we need to give him a gallon of mineral oil to lube him up so he can pass those worms," I said, as I shook the worms off onto the stall floor and removed the sleeve.

I reached for my stomach tube. "All right, Clifford, shorten up on his lead rope and hang on to his halter," I said. "Here we go." I slid one end of the stomach tube into Jeremiah's left nostril, down his esophagus, and into his stomach.

I REMEMBER WELL THE FIRST TIME I passed a stomach tube. I was pretty much just out of school and I had received an emergency call during the night to treat a colicky horse. I got everything ready, including a half gallon or so of mineral oil and warm water that I would pump into the horse's stomach once the tube was in place. I had the owner stand on one side of the horse hanging on to the halter while I stood on the other side. I then lubed up one end of the stomach tube and gently inserted it into the left nostril of the colicky horse.

"He's getting a bit of a nosebleed," the owner said to me as I began to pass the stomach tube down the horse's esophagus and into his stomach.

Nosebleeds from attempting to pass a nasogastric tube in a horse can be somewhat frightening when a horse owner sees one for the first time. There is often a lot of blood, and the bleeding can continue for a good twenty minutes. This particular horse owner likely knew, just as I did, that nosebleeds associated with attempts to pass a stomach tube are also a frequent complication of the neophyte veterinarian.

"I'm sure it will stop as soon as I take the tube out," I said.

"I hope so, but I've seen this happen before and usually they don't," the owner replied knowingly and somewhat sarcastically.

It was dark but I could see the blood puddling at the horse's feet. I administered the oil and water to the horse, withdrew the stomach tube, and told the owner that the horse should be fine by the morning.

"Hey, you're right, Doc, his nosebleed quit just as soon as you took the tube out," the owner said as he led the horse back to the stall.

"ALL RIGHT, GOOD NIGHT NOW," I said as I gathered up my gear and hurried back to my truck.

I climbed back inside the cab and turned the ignition

key. "Hey, Doc, wait a sec. Good job," the owner said.

Tears began to well up in my eyes. I was scared to look. I could feel the blood running down my arm and beginning to soak through my shirt. I drove out the driveway. Half a mile down the road I pulled over and flipped the lights on in the cab of the truck.

The end of my left thumb was crushed and the fingernail ripped fully off. It was dark when I was passing the stomach tube and somehow, as I inserted the tube in the horse's nostril, my thumb ended up between the horse's front teeth. The puddling blood by the horse's front feet was in fact my own, which of course was why I was able to reassure the owner that the "nosebleed" would stop as soon as I took the tube out.

"All right, Clifford, that oil will make it a lot easier for him to pass that ball of worms," I said as I withdrew the stomach tube.

I cleaned up my gear, headed back to the truck, and handed Clifford some deworming medication for Jeremiah.

"You'll need to keep an eye on him this evening but I think he'll be fine by the morning," I said. "And don't forget to give him that worming medicine tomorrow," I added as I got into my truck.

"You reckon I should put just a little more brake fluid down his ears just in case?" Clifford asked.

THE FIRST YEAR I SET UP PRACTICE IN CALIFORNIA, I had been called out on an emergency to examine a severely colicking horse. The abdominal pain was relentless and nonresponsive to any IV painkillers I administered. Although I had palpated the horse rectally to determine the source of the abdominal pain, I was unable to discover why the horse was colicking. I had the owners haul the horse three hours to a referral hospital for what I told them would be an expensive colic surgery to fix a likely twisted gut.

I contacted the surgeon while the horse was en route, and the surgeon in turn alerted the hospital staff that a surgical colic was arriving and to prep the operating room and ICU.

However, it wasn't very long after the horse arrived at the referral hospital that I received a call from the surgeon. "The horse is fine and ready to go back home," he told me.

"How can that be? Didn't he need colic surgery?" I asked, surprised to hear the dramatic news that the horse had improved so suddenly.

"Ear ticks was the problem," he responded. "We put a bit of tick medicine in both ears and sent the owners home with a couple-ounce squirt bottle in case it happens again."

THE COWBOYS OF CALIFORNIA knew about the severe muscle cramping and colic-like signs associated with an inner-ear tick infestation long before the symptoms were described in any equine veterinary textbook. Brake fluid was what was squirted down a colicky horse's ears before anyone ever called out a veterinarian.

Cowboys also knew that a pint of bourbon would cut the pain of a bellyachin' horse and that turpentine was a sure fix for bloat.

It was a couple of days later that I received a phone call from Clifford. "How's Jeremiah doing?" I asked.

"That wormin' medicine you left me worked real good," he answered. "The next day after I give it I ain't never seen such a pile a worms. I reckon them worms taken to resistin' tobacco juice."

"I got another problem though, Doc. It's Cupcake, and she got herself in a heap o' trouble. She done busted the stall door latch comin' out the stall in a hurry and gashed herself good. She's gonna need some stitchin' up," Clifford said. "I got her loaded in the trailer an' was thinkin' I could haul her over to your clinic and be there in 'bout an hour."

"That's fine, Clifford, bring her in. I'll see you when you get here," I replied.

As Clifford offloaded Cupcake from his trailer, I saw the bloody foot-long gash over her rib cage. "Problem is, Doc, I can't find the busted metal door latch. You reckon it might be inside her?"

"I'm not sure, but we'll know in just a couple of minutes. Bring her inside the exam room," I said.

Clifford led Cupcake into the exam room of the clinic. It was a good-size laceration that went deep into the muscles over her rib cage. I clipped and cleaned the wound with some betadine disinfect and infiltrated the wound edges with a local anesthetic. After probing the wound with some forceps I was unable to feel any part of the broken metal door latch.

I wheeled my ultrasound machine over to Cupcake. "I don't think it's in here, but I'm gonna scan her just to make sure," I said to Clifford.

Metallic foreign bodies are best detected by X-rays, but the portable X-ray machine I kept in the back of my vet truck was limited in its diagnostic capability and useful only for the legs and feet of horses. The giant-size X-ray machine that could see through the belly of a horse or a mule to find a buried piece of metal was something that hung from ceilings and was only to be found in universities and large referral hospitals.

My ultrasound machine, however, was high-tech, pricey, and I had gotten good at using it. It enabled me to become almost sleuth-like in being able to see the other side of something. I used it on mares to check for pregnancies and on horses' legs to evaluate tendon injuries. I scanned the bellies of colicky horses with it and used it to go looking for hematomas and abscesses that I thought might be lurking.

I knew that the image created by ultrasound waves bouncing off Cupcake's rib bones would appear the same as a piece of metal but I was savvy and clever and would be able to sort out rib from latch, based on size and location.

Clifford and I both stared closely at the screen of the ultrasound machine as I slowly moved the probe over the wound and in between Cupcake's ribs, looking for the buried and broken stall door latch.

"Nope, it's not in there," I said to Clifford as I turned off the ultrasound machine and brought out my suture tray and a pair of sterile gloves.

"Well, I reckon when she busted it off it must have fallen in the straw bedding, but I thought I done looked pretty good," Clifford responded.

The wound repair required a three-layer closure. I used absorbable catgut suture for the muscle and subcuticular layer and a polyethylene nonabsorbable for the overlying skin. "Nice job, Doc, you shoulda' been a seamstress," Clifford commented as I tied off the last skin suture.

"She's ready to go back home. Bring her back in a couple of weeks and I'll take the skin sutures out," I said, admiring the thirty or so sutures I had neatly and symmetrically placed.

Mules are smarter than horses but the expression "stubborn as a mule" has a real genetic basis. After suturing her up, we led Cupcake out of the exam room to the back of the trailer.

"Hang on, Doc," Clifford said. He handed me Cupcake's lead rope, walked to the front of the flatbed of his pickup truck, and unhooked a cable winch. He ran the metal cable through the front window of the two-horse trailer, out the back, and attached it to Cupcake's halter. Clifford then calmly walked back to the winch and ratcheted the mule onto the trailer. Cupcake never struggled, just leaned back and left a set of twenty-foot skid marks.

TWO WEEKS HAD GONE BY and Clifford had scheduled an appointment to have Cupcake's sutures removed.

I admired my suture work as he unloaded Cupcake from the trailer. "That healed up nicely," I said.

"Hang on, Doc, be right back. I got somethin' to show you," Clifford said after we led Cupcake into the exam room.

Clifford returned with one of those battery-operated, handheld, twenty-dollar-a-day rental items that people use on the beach to find loose change and lost rings. It was a metal detector.

"Never could find that busted stall door latch in Cupcake's stall. I reckoned it must have still been inside her," Clifford said as the beeping noise got progressively louder and more rapid as he moved the metal detector toward Cupcake's rib cage.

It was just a half-hour procedure to reopen the wound and remove the broken six-inch-long metal stall door latch that had migrated its way up from the muscle tissue to the underlying skin.

"I reckon I can guess how you got to being so good

with that needle and thread," Clifford commented as I tied the last knot.

"How's that?" I responded.

"Getting to stitch up the same wound twice is good practice," he answered with more than a bit of a smile.

It became somewhat of a "Do you remember when?" story that Clifford enjoyed bringing up more often than was to my liking over the years, one that left him chuckling and elbowing me in the ribs each time he told it.

{ELEVEN}

From Yank to Jackaroo

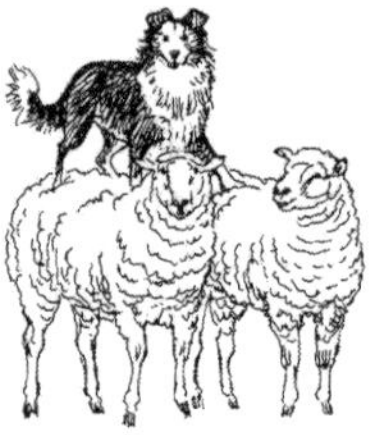

RANCHES IN AUSTRALIA ARE CALLED STATIONS, and I was the youngest of the five ranch hands, or "jackaroos," who worked on this particular sheep and cattle station in Western Australia. There was also a manager, an assistant manager, a bush mechanic, and a cook. Bush mechanic, by the way, is by no means a formal certification or licensure, it merely implies an inherent and perhaps somewhat uncanny ability to improvise when it comes to fixing stuff.

"Remote" would be an apt description of the location of the approximately eighty-thousand-acre sheep and cattle station I would work on for the next year of my life.

Water was sparse and windmills provided the power to pump water up from artesian wells for the livestock and ourselves. Mail was delivered once a week and it would be almost a year before I picked up a phone, read a newspaper, listened to a radio, or watched television. There were no power lines to provide electricity, refrigerators were kerosene powered, and our beer was homemade.

The sixty thousand or so sheep were Merinos, bred for their wool rather than their meat. Their wool is soft, warm and frequently blended with the likes of silk and cashmere in high-end performance athletic wear. Another desirable feature of the Merino sheep is its resilience and adaptability to inhospitable places like the interior scrub of Australia.

The three thousand head of cattle on the station were mostly Santa Gertrudis, a hardy Texas meat breed. Cattle are typically bred for their ability to produce either meat—the Angus or Hereford breeds, for example—or milk, for instance the Holstein or Jersey breeds. Santa Gertrudis cattle are a tropical breed of cattle developed on the King Ranch in Texas and known for their ability to adjust well to harsh climates.

My first day on the station would be a memorable one. I hopped out of the Land Rover, dropped my gear off at the bunkhouse, and went out to meet the other jackaroos who had mustered into the yards a flock of ewes that had recently lambed.

It was an assembly-line procedure of sorts, in which the lambs were caught up and placed upside down in a rotating device called a lamb cradle. I watched impressed as two jackaroos were busy catching up the lambs and placing them in the cradle while another two jackaroos were docking and castrating.

As each week-old lamb was placed on the cradle, a jackaroo would dock its tail. If it happened to be a ram lamb, the jackaroo would also cut off the tip of the scrotal sac to expose the testicles, lean down, and deftly grab both testicles with his teeth and with a quick yank, spit both testicles out onto a growing pile already on the ground.

Smiling and with blood smeared around his mouth, one of the jackaroos turned to welcome me: "You must be the Yank we've been hearing about. You ready to get to work, mate?"

The next year of my life would be challenging, arduous, and wonderfully fun. The days would begin with chores before daylight, and following breakfast the day's real work started.

Two dairy cows had to be milked by hand daily, a chore agreeably allotted to the youngest jackaroo. Sunshine and Massy were kind-eyed Jersey cows and for the most part quite forgiving of someone who had never milked a cow before. Massy had been through a couple of bouts of mastitis, which presumably is how she came by her name. Only two of the four teats of her udder "worked." Nonetheless, she gave what she could, which was usually not much more than half a gallon a day.

Both cows enjoyed the routine. They were there waiting for me to let them into the milking shed at five thirty each morning. I'd slide the shed door open and they'd walk over to their stanchions and find the grain in the manger.

Cow manure and horse manure differ primarily in their consistency. When cows poop, it plops and splatters. Sitting on a stool by a cow's udder before daybreak retrieving more than just the occasional fleck of manure from out of the milking pail is philosophically a bit like much of life, a reminder that life isn't perfect and humor is helpful.

"Chooks" is Aussie lingo for chickens, and chooks' eggs and mutton liver is what we usually had for breakfast. The cook served up our plates of food covered with fly netting, something like cheesecloth. The ever-present blowflies would otherwise do a "fly by," dropping maggots on the food.

Mutton is sheep meat, and the older crippled-up sheep were put in a killer pen from which we butchered two every Friday. The hung carcasses were cut up on Saturday as chops, ribs, and roasts and portioned out to the manager, assistant manager, mechanic, and of course the cook who prepared all the meals for the five jackaroos.

Life on the farm, or "station," I should say, was very much one of self-sufficiency. Catching in a pen and butchering what I would eat the next week was an opportunity for reflection. There was no grocer's meat case from which one could toss a one-pound package of ground chuck into a grocery cart and no dairy aisle where one could reach for a quart of milk. Every fortnight we got paid and a pint or two of Swan lager at the local pub was an eighty-mile drive along dirt roads.

It would take several lonely months before I really became a jackaroo in the eyes of the others I worked alongside. I suppose it was really a time of testing to see if I had what it took to be one of them. There seemed to just come a day when I was brought into the fold, taken in so to speak, a time when I was no longer "the Yank" but rather just the youngest jackaroo.

I recall on several occasions while herding cattle on horseback in the scrub we would see an emu or a big red kangaroo. As a bit of diversionary entertainment, I would slip away from the cattle drive and give chase. A five-foot-tall emu can outrun any horse, and a big red "roo" can outmaneuver even the zippiest steed. It was always a futile but nonetheless very fun game of chase that the other jackaroos smilingly dismissed as lingering adolescence on my part.

At the end of most days a mob of wallabies could be seen grazing at dusk. I raised an orphan joey kangaroo in a pillowcase that I hung from a doorknob in the bunkhouse. The mechanic had raised one that lived in his front yard, and every so often it would disappear for a few days into the bush and then return. Gone "walkabout," something that in some respects I was doing with my own life.

I worked in the wool shed with the thirty or so Aborigines who spent six weeks on the station shearing the thousands of sheep. Sadly, discrimination against the indigenous Australians, the Aborigines, was a reality. They were prejudicially referred to as "abos" and "black fellas" and were not only forbidden to ride up front in the cab of the farm pickups, but relegated to "the back of the bus" in any number of other ways.

Hadley was invaluable. He was an Aussie sheepdog and by himself he could muster a "mob" of five or six hundred sheep through a gated paddock. When hundreds of sheep were brought into the yards for vaccines and deworming, it was Hadley that ran up and down their backs to "tighten up the mob" in the chutes.

December in the Southern hemisphere is a summer month, and Christmas Day was searing hot. Rather than leave me to spend Christmas by myself after the other jackaroos had left for a couple of days to see family for the holiday, the manager stopped by the bunkhouse in the Land Rover. We drove through twenty miles of scrub and arrived on a bluff overlooking a magnificent stretch of West Australian beach. Wading out amidst the shallows of the Indian Ocean with rod and reel, we spent the day surfcasting for skipjack and spotted mackerel.

Tall, tanned, and rugged, the manager was from Katoomba, a town in the Blue Mountains where the rock formations are canyon-like and spectacular. He was dressed in khaki and wore a brimmed canvas hat with a chin cord. He would have been my dad's age, and as we stood in the shallows side by side I sensed my dad would have smiled knowing how I spent that Christmas Day.

The manager taught me how to use the snake-bite kit. He also told me to walk carefully when near a creek bed where one of the most venomous snakes in the world, the tiger snake, was likely to be found escaping the heat of the day.

MY YEAR IN THE OUTBACK OF WESTERN AUSTRALIA would change my life. I would come to appreciate the value of hard work and develop a love for the outdoors and its extraordinary wildlife. I also came to respect the speed of a one-ton Santa Gertrudis bull as it turned to charge a not-so-knowing young jackaroo on horseback. And it was in Australia that I first worked with a veterinarian who encouraged me to pursue a career in the wonderful world of veterinary medicine.

{TWELVE}

Angel Slippers

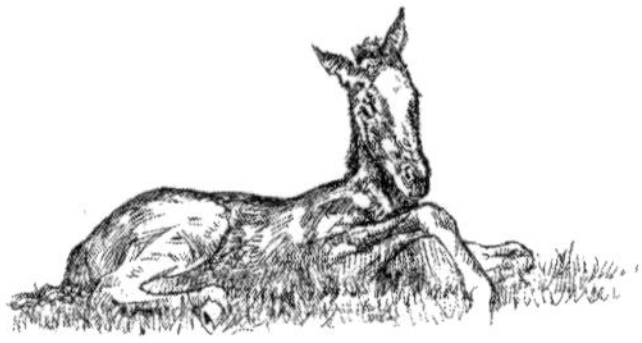

IT WAS A FRIDAY IN EARLY SPRING and close on midnight as I reached for my cell phone on the night table.

"Hey, Doc, it's me, Paul. I'm sorry to be calling so late but I got a five-year-old maiden that's having a bit of trouble foaling," he said, sounding a little out of breath. "She's got the white sac showing and she's been pushing pretty hard, but I don't see the foal coming," he added.

"All right, Paul, I'll be there in forty-five minutes," I replied, hopping out of bed.

I was out the front door and in my vet truck within ten minutes.

Paul was the manager of an Arabian horse farm in San Simeon, a small coastal town in central California. The owners were prominent in the publishing of newspapers and magazines, built a mansion as big as a castle, and owned fourteen miles of Pacific coast along Highway 1.

The forty or so horses were Polish Arabians and the farm

was located along the ocean, past a bridge and down a small dirt road lined with giant eucalyptus trees and coastal pines.

The barns were surrounded by manicured gardens of ferns, rhododendrons, and magnolias, and the paddocks overlooked flower-filled coastal bluffs stretching out to the sea. The architecture of the stables was Spanish and Mediterranean, the buildings white with stucco archways, and the roofs of red tile. It was everything *Town & Country* and *House Beautiful,* all seemingly simple yet elegant, provincial and yet *Cosmopolitan.*

SITTING ON THE FENCE OF A BROODMARE PADDOCK in spring watching the mares graze will make you smile. The pregnant belly of a mare heavy with foal seems to—and in fact does—have a life of its own. "Wow, there's a lot of running around going on in there," you might say to yourself, surprised by the late-gestation fetal movement.

A horse veterinarian does a lot of thinking and worrying on the way to a mare having trouble foaling. It's not at all like casually doing a lameness exam midmorning or chit-chatting one's way through the afternoon while vaccinating a barnful of horses. It's a true emergency where minutes make a difference if the mare and foal are to have a chance at surviving.

Ninety percent of mares foal between midnight and five in the morning. If all goes as it should, it wouldn't make any difference if anyone was there or not. Everything happens in less than twenty minutes. The mare breaks a sweat, her cervix dilates, and as she bears down and squeezes, one of the two placental sacs ruptures at the cervical opening, causing a gush of placental fluid to spill to the outside.

Within just a few minutes of the mare breaking her

water, the foal's head and legs appear at the mare's vulva, covered by the smoky-gray amnionic sac. After almost a year of gestation, it's done, that's it. The foal stands within one hour, nurses within two hours, and the mare passes her placenta within three hours after foaling. In fact, that's the "one-two-three rule" of foaling and it's just about that easy . . . most of the time.

What really is remarkable is that minutes before birth, the foal is completely in the wrong position to be born. If you had X-ray vision and looked at a mare heavy with foal in the last few months of her gestation, you would see the foal lying upside down on its back along the curve of the mare's belly. An attempted delivery with the foal in this position would be disastrous and would likely result in the loss of both the mare and the foal.

Amazingly enough, the complex cascade of hormones during labor signals the foal to "wake up" and rotate itself right side up. This rotational positioning is essential for a normal delivery and occurs just minutes prior to birth. After twisting to right itself, the foal then passes through the birth canal, its head between its forelegs, one shoulder slightly in back of the other to help minimize the space needed to pass through the mare's pelvic canal.

To assist with the corkscrew-type maneuver the foal needs to perform in order to correctly position itself before birth, the mare somehow senses what needs to be done and tries to help. A mare in labor will frequently stand up, lay back down, then pace the stall, often looking at her flanks almost as if to see if the foal has managed to turn itself.

To the inexperienced observer, this up-and-down behavior, coupled with the mare's pacing and sometimes even rolling, seems cause for alarm. Impatience is what you might feel as you wonder, "What is she doing? Why is she getting up and down? Is she colicking? And why doesn't she just lie down and push?" The mare, however, is actually trying to help the foal twist and rotate into the correct position to be born.

IT WAS DIFFICULT TO SEE BUT WONDERFUL TO SMELL. The coastal fog had come in off the ocean late that afternoon, and driving along the Pacific on Highway 1 at close on one in the morning was slow. I rolled down the window and knew I was getting close. The salt smell of the air was cool, moist, and mint-like from the groves of giant eucalyptus trees I was passing.

I crossed the Pico Creek Bridge, turned down the dirt road, and saw the lights on in the broodmare barn.

I hopped out of my truck, taking with me my grip from behind the seat as well as the large aluminum case that contained obstetrical equipment. I saw Paul and Big Juan, who usually worked in the yearling barn, standing outside one of the stalls halfway down the barn aisle. "Hey, Doc, she's in here. We just got done walking her."

"Hi, Paul, how's she doing, any change?" I asked.

"No, nothing different," Paul said as he slid open the stall door and snapped the lead rope onto her leather halter.

"*Hola*, Juan, good to see you," I said.

"*Usted tambien*," Juan replied.

I walked up to the bay mare and stroked her sweat-drenched neck and shoulder. It was easy to see from her eye, she was worried. "Good girl, it'll be all right," I said, noticing the brass nameplate on the cheek strap of her halter: Gipsy Maid.

"How long you think she's been pushing?" I asked.

"I pretty much know exactly just how long it's been—coming up close on two hours. Juan was doing the foal watch and happened to be walking by her stall when she broke her water. I came up from the house as soon as he called me. The white sac is all there's been. She's been up and down, groaning, and pushing up a storm," Paul said.

"Is she close on her due date?" I asked.

"Yup, she's right at 343 days from her last breeding date," Paul replied.

I stepped behind the mare, pulled her wrapped tail to the side, and saw just what Paul had described: only the smoky-gray amnionic sac.

"Watch it, Doc, I think she's wanting to go down," Paul said, slapping her on the shoulder to stop her from trying to go down.

"Keep her up, Paul, I'll be right back."

I quickly stepped outside the stall, knelt down, opened my grip, and grabbed a syringe and a vial of medication to sedate her. "Here we go, Paul," I said, holding off the mare's jugular and slipping a needle into her vein. I attached the syringe and pushed. "That will sedate her for a bit," I said.

"Paul, can you round up a couple of buckets of hot water and a bunch of towels," I asked.

"I'm a step ahead of ya, Doc. Everything's right here," he said.

Using a couple of handfuls of water-soaked cotton and some betadine disinfect, I cleaned up Gipsy Maid's perineal area then rolled up my left sleeve.

"Paul, you got her?" I asked.

"Yeah, Doc, she's looking pretty out of it."

"Hang on, here we go," I said, lubing up my arm with

some soapy disinfect. I tore the amnionic sac open and passed my hand into her vagina. I should have immediately felt the foal's front legs outstretched and in front but I didn't. Sliding my hand beyond her cervix and into her uterus, I felt the foal's head and forelegs flexed at the knees.

"Whadda ya think, Doc?" Paul asked anxiously.

Just then, Gipsy Maid groaned as she started to bear down, squeezing my arm back out. "Hang on a sec, Paul, I gotta come out. She's pushing pretty hard." I withdrew my arm and waited for her to stop straining.

"Let me go again. You ready?" I said. I lubed up my arm and passed it back through the torn sac. I had just enough time to check what I needed to know before Gipsy Maid began to strain again. I pinched the foal's forearm and felt it reflexively twitch. The foal was still alive.

I withdrew my arm and found a towel. "Paul, here's what's going on," I said. "She can push all day, that foal is stuck. It's a bilateral carpal flexion, but good news is, it's alive."

"It's a what?" Paul asked.

"The foal's forelegs are flexed; they're bent at the knees and up against the brim of her pelvis. It'll never make it through the birth canal. She'll push, prolapse, tear and rupture everything before the foal comes out."

"What do we do?" Paul asked. "Should we send her to the clinic for a C-section?"

"It's three hours away. We'll lose the foal if we ship her," I answered. "It's alive now but won't be for too much longer. Problem is, I can't straighten the legs out to get them up and over into the birth canal with her straining like she is. I have to be able to push the foal back into the uterus and then see if I can bring those legs up. It will hopefully only take twenty minutes to do and we'll need everyone's help."

"All right, Doc, let's go for it. What do you want us to do?"

"Juan, there's a coiled-up rope behind the passenger seat of my truck. Can you grab it?" I asked. "Paul, here's the game plan. We'll need to get a catheter in quick. We could try an epidural to stop her from straining, but I don't think that will be enough. I'm going to need you to give her some medication while I'm working on the other end."

I quickly scrubbed up the area over Gipsy Maid's jugular vein with some disinfect and a few squirts of alcohol.

I knelt down beside the big aluminum box containing my obstetrical gear. Inside was another smaller case with catheters of all sizes. I opened it up and took out a five-inch, large-bore, 14-gauge catheter.

"Doc, that looks like a harpoon," Paul commented as I held off Gipsy Maid's jugular vein again and waited for the vein to distend. "We may need to give her several injections before we're done and probably some fluids later. When she needs more meds, you'll be giving them through the catheter, as I'll be busy on the other end," I said as I slipped the five-inch needle into her jugular and waited for blood to flash back in the hub. I was in. I advanced the needle a bit farther then slid the five-inch Teflon catheter down and off the needle into the vein. I capped the catheter and then threw in a couple of whip stitches with some suture to secure it in place.

"Here you go, Doc, I found it," Juan said, returning from my truck and laying the cotton rope on the floor outside the stall.

"Thanks. We're almost ready. I just need to mix up a few syringes."

Kneeling down by my grip, I took out the necessary vials of Rompun, Valium, and Torb to make up a couple of syringes of IV triple cocktails and ketamine to follow.

AFTER GRADUATING FROM VETERINARY SCHOOL, I spent the following year as an intern at the veterinary college at Ohio State University. One of the school's clients was a large Standardbred horse farm with eight stallions and over three hundred mares. During that particular breeding season, more than two hundred mares were due to foal in a two-month span.

I spent my days working in the university's large-animal clinics and my nights in the farm's foaling barns. The foaling crew knew to rouse me from my naps on the office sofa when they found a mare in labor. There was much watching and waiting during those late-night hours, but there was also much to be learned and gained in the sorting-out of what was normal and what wasn't. I managed to watch over 150 mares foal in that two-month period and began to develop a sense of when things were going as they should and when the mare was going to need help.

I worked with a professor in equine obstetrics who taught me much. In the labor and delivery room of a foaling stall, late at night, we were alongside a mare having trouble foaling. I was there to learn, he to teach, and our shared objective was to save both mare and foal. "Time is trauma, time is trauma," he would say, reprimanding me as I stood bare-armed, up to my shoulder inside a mare. "C'mon, c'mon, get in and get out, quit mucking around in there," he would continue as I struggled blindly to sort out by feel the obstetrical dilemma of a foal unable to be born.

The mare doesn't instinctually recognize the fact that

if her foal is positioned incorrectly, it can't be born. She is incapable of knowing that the foal with the flexed knees can't pass through the birth canal until the legs are straightened or that the foal with the turned neck can't pass until the neck is brought round right.

Powerful uterine contractions exerted against a malpositioned foal merely result in greater tissue swelling and the foal becoming further impacted or "stuck." The swelling and edema result in narrowing of a birth canal where the margin for anything but perfect doesn't exist. Complicating the dilemma of a mare with a malpositioned foal is her instinctual response to push. Panic-driven, the mare frantically pushes against a trapped foal that can't enter the birth canal. The relentless heaving tragically results in a fatal prolapse, hemorrhage, and rupture.

These same forceful uterine contractions by the mare also impair a veterinary obstetrician's ability to efficiently determine what part of the foal is causing the impasse. As the veterinarian moves their arm forward beyond the vaginal canal into the uterus to assess the malpositioned foal, waves of contractions exerted by the mare push in opposition. The sorting-out by blind feel which part of the foal is not correctly positioned for birth must be performed quickly, between contractions, and without further trauma to the mare.

On countless foaling emergencies late at night, I recall standing pressed up against a panicky mare's back legs with one arm shoulder-deep into her uterus feeling placenta-covered jumbled limbs. I often would momentarily close my eyes to shut out the rest of the world, to try and make sense of what I was feeling. "Am I holding a front leg or a back leg?" "Where's the foal's head?" "Am I feeling the side of the shoulder or a hip?" "Can I pinch some skin to see if it is still alive?" "Do these legs belong to just one foal or is there a twin?"

"Paul, we gotta drop her," I said.

"Okay, Doc", he responded, just a bit unsure if he'd heard me right. "You mean just lay her down in the stall, right here, right now, before we get the baby out?" he asked.

"We can't get the baby out unless we knock her out," I said. "I could give her an epidural to stop the straining but it wouldn't give me any more room to straighten out those front legs. If we drop her and hoist up her hind legs, everything in her belly will sort of slide forward. I can push the baby back in her belly, giving me enough room to bring the foal's front legs up and over. Hopefully we'll only need to keep her out for twenty minutes. I'll need Juan's help with the rope and you may have to give her more of the anesthesia if we need more time," I explained.

Paul held on to Gipsy Maid as I slipped a needle through the rubber injection cap of the catheter. "I've made up another couple syringes for you to give her if we need more time," I said to Paul as I attached the syringe containing the IV triple cocktail and pushed.

In less than a minute Gipsy Maid had her nose almost to the stall floor and began to sway back and forth. "She's ready for the ketamine, which will drop her," I said to Paul. I inserted a needle through the injection cap, attached the syringe full of ketamine, and pushed.

"Let me have her until she goes down," I said, taking the lead rope from Paul. As Gipsy Maid started to slowly buckle, I directed her fall so she would be lying down with the catheter side up and accessible.

"Paul, here's the second set of syringes. Watch the time

and stay by her head," I said. I placed a towel over Gipsy Maid's eyes. "We'll have about twenty minutes or so before we need to give her more. If you see her ears start to twitch, she's thinking about waking up," I said.

"Juan, *por favor amigo*, I need your help. Can you toss one end of the rope over that truss?" I asked. "You're going to need to pull as I lift."

I looped a couple of half hitches over each of Gipsy Maid's lower hind legs. We worked quickly and in unison, pulling, hoisting, and managing to lift her haunches up off the ground by almost a foot. Fortunately, Gipsy Maid, being an Arabian, was a lighter-framed horse than, say, a beefy-ended Quarter horse or a heavy warmblood.

The idea was to raise her haunches up off the ground enough so that the foal would slide forward in Gipsy Maid's belly. The flexed front legs of the foal would then no longer be right up against the brim of the bony birth canal. The mare would also be unconscious and therefore unable to strain against my attempts to push the foal back away from her pelvis. With a little luck, I might have just enough room to straighten the foal's legs and position them in the birth canal.

Time was critical. The placenta, which functions in part to deliver oxygen to the unborn, quickly begins to separate from the wall of the uterus after the mare breaks her water and goes into labor. Gipsy Maid's foal was already likely starting to suffocate.

"Here we go. Juan, hang on to that rope, and Paul, watch the time and her ears," I said as I lubed up my arms with some soapy disinfect.

I slid one arm quickly into the mare's vagina, past her cervix, and into her uterus. The foal had indeed slid back and away from the mare's pelvis. I was between the mare's back legs, shoulder-deep, blindly following my way down one of the foal's forearms to where I was able to grasp the cannon bone. "All right, Paul, I've got a leg. Let me see if I can straighten it out," I said and slowly and carefully pulled the flexed front leg out in front of the foal.

"How's our time, Paul?" I asked.

"Almost twelve minutes now and her ears aren't moving," Paul answered.

"All right, that's good. We're halfway there. Juan, you okay with the rope?"

I ran my hand down the forearm of the other leg and grasped the foal's cannon bone.

I managed to straighten the foal's other flexed leg only partially before feeling some resistance. I hesitated to pull more. I knew the resistance I felt was the foal's hoof dragging along the wall of the uterus. I decided to wait a few moments and recalled the words of warning from my obstetrics professor about what I was trying to do. He had reminded me of the fact that because the limbs of the unborn foal are as long as its mother's, there is significant risk of causing a uterine tear to the mare while trying to straighten the flexed forelimbs of a malpositioned foal. A torn uterus would be my fault and would require belly surgery for Gipsy Maid at a referral center.

It's somehow odd to think that the legs of a newborn foal are as long as its mother's. Yet, as the opening paragraph of any anatomy book is likely to emphasize, structure and function are purposefully linked, and a newborn foal at only two days old can gallop alongside its mother.

"Hey, Paul, you're gonna have to give her another set of syringes. She's gotta relax more," I said.

"Gotcha, Doc, will do," Paul responded, and he soon announced, "It's done, Doc. She got 'em."

"Good, let's give it half a minute to kick in." I came back out of the mare and lubed up my arm again with more soapy disinfect.

"Juan, you still okay hanging on to that rope?" I asked.

"I'm good, Doc. I got it."

Big Juan was just that, big and also strong. He was from Mexico, worked with the yearlings keeping the sometimes rambunctious colts and fillies in line, and helped with the mares during foaling season.

"Ready to go again, you guys?" I said as I slid my arm back into the mare's uterus, feeling to find the remaining flexed foreleg of the foal.

The muscle-relaxing properties of Valium on the mare's myometrium, the muscular layer of the uterus, was what I was after. This sheet of muscle needed to relax a bit more to allow me some stretch, so I could pull the foal's leg around without tearing the mare's uterus.

I grasped the cannon bone of the remaining flexed front leg of the foal and pulled. "Okay, okay, that's good," I said out loud as I pulled a bit more and suddenly felt the resistance lessen. "I think we got it," I said. "Lower her down, Juan. We're good."

Both front legs of the foal were now out in front, in a dive-like position in the birth canal, where they were supposed to have been almost three hours ago when the mare went into labor. "C'mon, give me a hand, Juan, and grab a leg. Ready, pull."

We pulled the foal out onto the straw, toweling off its face and clearing its nostrils. The foal gasped and its eyes opened. I rubbed its chest with the towel and it gave out a little nicker. Gipsy Maid heard her foal, raised her towel-covered head, and although still a little woozy from the anesthesia, managed a nicker back.

I had Juan remove the ropes from Gipsy Maid's legs while I went for my stethoscope to have a listen on the baby. I knelt down by the foal and placed my stethoscope over its chest. The heart rate was steady, no murmurs, and the lungs sounded clear. As I continued to listen, my eyes followed the foal's legs down to its hooves and I smiled. There they were—"angel slippers," the rubbery, gelatinous, sneaker-like "shoes" that cover each of the sharp-ended, pointy hooves of the unborn foal.

Angel slippers . . . They dry up and disappear within a day after a foal is born, so you may never have had a chance to see them, but surely they are aptly named. They come standard as a safety feature on the not-yet-born foal and serve to protect the mare's reproductive tract from bruising, scrapes, and perforations by the sometimes rambunctious activity of a wanna-be-born foal. Surely, they also helped prevent an inadvertent uterine tear as I straightened out the foal's flexed forelimbs.

"Doc, we got it from here, we know what to do," Paul said. "We'll make sure the foal gets to nursing, and I'll save the placenta for you to take a look at tomorrow."

"All right, Paul, let me pull the catheter from the mare and I'll see you in the morning. Hey, Juan, *gracias amigo*," I said as I rounded up my gear.

"De nada, Doc, hasta mañana."

I was tired and it was late. I would have to come back in the morning to check on the baby. I was heading down the barn aisle back to the truck when Paul called out, "Hey, Doc!" I turned around. "Don't you want to know?" he asked. He saw my puzzled expression. "It's a filly!"

{THIRTEEN}

Out of the Starting Gate

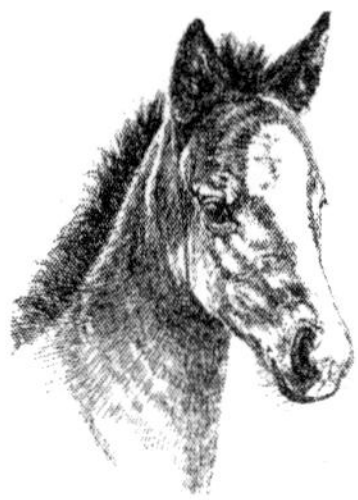

IT WAS LATE THE NEXT MORNING and I was back to check on Gipsy Maid's filly. I parked outside the broodmare barn, hopped out of the truck, grabbed my grip from behind the seat, and headed into the barn.

Paul was standing outside Gipsy Maid's stall. "Hey, Doc, good to see ya," he said.

"How's the filly?" I asked.

"Well, perhaps not as good as I had hoped. I'm a bit worried 'bout her," Paul said. "Something's not right. She's not nursing on her own and she walks around like she's not sure where she's going, almost like she can't see so good."

"What do you mean?" I asked.

"Well, it seems she wants to nurse, but it's like she can't find the faucet and hook on. We've been milking out the mare and bottle-feeding her every couple of hours but problem is, milk gets to running out her nose when we do."

"Let me watch her a bit," I said to Paul. We stood

outside the stall and observed Gipsy Maid and her filly. The mare seemed to have bounced back from the night before. She was bright and alert, eating her hay, and I could see she had passed several piles of manure during the night. The water was down in her buckets, which meant she was drinking. This was all good and I would have a closer look at her later.

In the meantime, what Paul said about Gipsy Maid's newborn filly was true. The filly seemed a bit out of it, and although I could understand why Paul thought she couldn't see so well, I suspected that something else was wrong.

"I agree with you, Paul. Something's not right," I said. The filly wasn't as bright and playful as a newborn foal should be but instead seemed almost depressed and uninterested in both her surroundings and the mare.

"Will she try to nurse on her own?" I asked Paul.

"Well, she'll kinda wander over to the mare as if she's thinking 'bout it but then it's as if she doesn't know what to do," Paul replied.

As we waited and watched from outside the stall, I saw what Paul had described. The filly would walk toward the mare as if she wanted to nurse but instead of turning and positioning her head to nurse, she would simply bump the mare's udder with her head. Of course, the milk let-down reflex of the mare was stimulated by the foal doing this, which resulted in the streaming of milk from Gipsy Maid's teats. The foal, however, just stood under the mare's udder, almost as if she were in a daze, seemingly oblivious to the near cascade of milk flowing down her face and muzzle. "See what I mean, Doc, she ain't right at all. Whadda ya think?" Paul asked.

"Let's catch her up," I said to Paul and slid the stall

door open. Gipsy Maid raised her head from her hay to have a look as we walked toward her filly. "The mare's good, Doc, not to worry," Paul commented. He closed the stall door behind him and the mare put her head back down to munch some more hay.

What Paul meant by reassuring me that the mare was "good" had to do with the fact that not all mares with newborns at their side are as accommodating as Gipsy Maid was about having us come in the stall with her foal. Many a mare can be so maternally protective that to walk into their stall can be somewhat of a precarious undertaking.

Veterinarians are understandably cautious about going in a stall to catch up and examine a newborn foal. There are mares that respond to a quiet voice and a reassuring way and are more trusting about having their foals approached. And then there are those that make quite clear the imminent peril involved in even considering entering the stall. These are the mares that, with ears pinned, rush to rake their teeth along the grillwork of the stall door as soon as the veterinarian enters the barn. The post-foaling exam is understandably rather brief with these mares and is wisely limited to a diagnostic glance from outside the stall to assess that both mare and foal are healthy.

Paul quietly walked up to the filly and effortlessly restrained her for me to examine. The ease with which he was able to do so was already cause for concern, as ordinarily catching a healthy newborn foal can be a bit of a rodeo. Even at only twenty-four-hours old a foal has a pretty good buck in them. They can be feisty, quick with a kick, and not at all cooperative about being restrained for the physical exam and blood draw. In fact, if there is a time when the job description most befitting a horse vet seems to be both a construction worker and a pediatrician, it would be while working with foals. One wouldn't think that a foal could get up much speed in the confines of a stall or instinctively know how to buck and kick at such an early age. But they can and do, and they're actually pretty good at it.

Gipsy Maid's foal was a dainty bay filly with a small white star on her forehead and a right hind stocking. She made no attempt to struggle as Paul held her for me to examine, but remained unusually quiet. There was something more than her being simply depressed or weak, a lack of awareness about her, a sort of not knowing. As I knelt down beside her, I stroked her shoulder and used my voice to reassure her that we were there to help. She was much too quiet for what should have been a bouncy and feisty Arabian filly.

Her gums were pink but a bit too dry, her eyes clear, and her capillary refill time somewhat delayed. Because Paul had mentioned that when they bottle-fed her, milk would reflux out her nose, I carefully examined the back of the filly's mouth to rule out the possibility of her having a cleft palate. I checked her temperature and that was normal, then passed my hand under her belly to feel her umbilicus so I could rule out the presence of an infection or hernia. Next I pinched a bit of skin over her shoulder and after letting go, watched to see how quickly the skin snapped back. It was a simple procedure called a skin tent test. If the pinched or tented-up skin failed to return quickly to its normal position, which was the case with Gipsy Maid's filly, this would indicate that she was dehydrated.

The degree of dehydration was mild to moderate and almost to be anticipated as the filly had yet to nurse on her own. Attempts to bottle-feed the filly once every couple of hours weren't working all that well and were also somewhat worrisome because of the nasal reflux. Milk refluxing out the filly's nostrils when she was bottle-fed meant that the nerves and muscles involved in the swallow reflex weren't fully functioning. Milk that wasn't being swallowed could also just as easily run down her windpipe into her lungs, causing an aspiration pneumonia.

"Don't you think she's a bit too quiet?" Paul asked.

"I agree. Let me have a bit of a listen on her," I said, and I took out my stethoscope from my grip. I had listened to the filly's chest shortly after she was born and had found that her heartbeat was regular, there were no murmurs, and her lungs sounded clear. Again, all sounded good, but I continued to listen to the filly's chest, using the moments to gather my thoughts, to pull together the pieces of the puzzle of all that had happened with Gipsy Maid's filly, and to decide how best to treat her.

"How's she sound, Doc?" Paul asked, as I took my stethoscope off.

"Her heart and lungs sound good," I replied.

"I was worried for a bit. Seemed like you were listening almost a bit too long."

I had a pretty good idea what was wrong. Paul was right, the filly did seem dazed, almost in a stupor, and in all likelihood it was from the traumatic birth the night before.

"Let her go, Paul, and let's see what she does," I said. Paul and I watched as the filly wandered over into a corner of the stall, where for several moments she would press her head against the wall. "Ay, you see that, Doc? What's wrong with her?" Paul asked.

The filly's inability to nurse and aimless wandering about the stall was characteristic of a type of dementia seen in traumatized foals. Her clumsy behavior and apparent blindness suggested damage to her delicate nervous system had occurred during her difficult birth.

Lost in thought and wondering if there was anything I could have done differently the night before to help prevent what had happened to the filly, I heard Paul say, "Doc, whadda ya think? Is there something we can do?"

"Paul, here's what is going on," I said. "Last night, we may not have gotten the filly out soon enough. We tried, but the mare's placenta probably separated before we could get the filly out to breathe on her own.

"There's something that happens in children that's kind of similar to what happened with this filly. Have you ever heard of cerebral palsy in kids?" I asked.

"Ay, somethin' wrong with their brain," he replied.

"You're right. It's usually associated with a lack of oxygen to the brain around the time of birth and results in some degree of lost muscle tone and coordination," I explained.

"You mean the filly is retarded, sort of like them 'dummy foals' I've heard about?" Paul asked.

"Not really so much retarded as her muscle coordination and movement are affected," I replied.

"But we did everything we could last night," Paul said.

"Thanks, I think we did too," I replied.

"So do we put her down?" Paul asked.

"Not yet. There's a chance that just because she's a bit slow coming out of the starting gate doesn't mean she can't still win the race."

"What do you mean? You think she might come round right?" Paul asked hopefully.

"We'll know in a few days, but it's going to take some work and we'll need some extra help," I responded.

"We got lots of barn help during the day and Juan's

doing the foal watch at night, so he can give a hand. Whadda ya want us to do?" Paul asked.

"Good, let's get to work and give it a go," I said. "If you'll round up a stable blanket and a halter for the filly, I'll grab some gear from my truck."

The dazed and dementia-like behavior of Gipsy Maid's filly was characteristic of a condition known as neonatal maladjustment syndrome, a disorder in fact quite similar to cerebral palsy in infants. The term "dummy foals" is somewhat misleading, however, in that the use of the word "dummy" suggests a lack of intelligence, as in a person who is mentally retarded. Yet this is not the case at all. What is lost to some degree in both cerebral palsy and neonatal maladjustment syndrome are motor skills, purposeful movement, and coordination. The etiology, or cause, is often associated with birth trauma or delayed delivery resulting in hypoxic injury to the delicate nerve tissue of the brain.

Infants with diminished blood oxygen around the time of birth who go on to develop cerebral palsy suffer permanent brain damage, much like an elderly person who has experienced a stroke. Both old and young suffer the same type of devastating injury from diminished oxygen to the brain. Impaired motor skills, loss of muscle movement and coordination all result from hypoxic injury to the brain. Tragically, because nervous tissue has no ability to regenerate, neurons that are lost or damaged remain so.

Oddly enough, however, in foals there is something rather unique about their nervous system. Although, as in humans, injured nervous tissue doesn't have the capacity to regenerate or grow back, in foals the damaged neurons seem to be more resilient to varying types of trauma than those of human infants. The unique ability of the foal's nervous system to somehow bounce back from the potentially devastating effects of cerebral hypoxia was my hope with Gipsy Maid's filly.

"Here ya go, Doc, where do you want it?" Paul asked, holding the stable blanket.

"Let's take it in the stall and lay it right here on the straw," I said. I brought in my grip and placed it on the blanket.

"All right, little one, here we go," I said, as I picked up the filly and gently laid her on her side on the blanket.

"That was a bit too easy, Doc, she didn't struggle none," Paul said.

Gipsy Maid turned her head to have a look at what we were doing and to make sure that her filly was okay.

Paul and I knelt over the filly as she lay all too quietly on her side on the blanket, and I began to scrub up her neck with some betadine disinfect. "All right, let's see what we can do for her. I'll need your help mixing up some medications and keeping her still in case she tries to move," I said, placing a catheter in her jugular vein.

The filly would need fluids, electrolytes, and anti-inflammatory IV meds over the next few days. She would also need an IV liter or two of antibody-rich plasma, as she likely didn't receive enough colostrum, or "first milk," within the first six to eight hours after being born.

Fortunately, nasogastric tubes—stomach tubes—come in all different sizes for horses, including ones small enough to use in foals. Because the filly had lost at least in part her ability to swallow, she would need to have a stomach tube left in place for the next few days. Paul and Juan could administer mare's milk through the feeding tube directly into the filly's stomach without the risks involved in bottle-feeding her and having milk end up in her lungs.

"All right, Paul, I think we're good. Let's get some fluids running to her," I said as I hooked up an IV line to a liter of Ringer's solution. "Open it up and let it run. She'll be needing at least three or four more liters in the next three hours. I'll be right back. I gotta get some more stuff from the truck." I left Paul holding the liter bag of electrolyte solution above her head.

I returned with a couple more liters of Ringer's solution, to one of which I had added 100 cc of DMSO. "How's she doing, Paul?" I asked as I laid the bags of fluids on the blanket.

"Good. She's just been laying here real quiet," Paul replied.

"She's gonna smell sort of funny in a bit," I told him as I changed the near empty liter bag he had been holding with the one containing DMSO.

"Whadda ya mean?" he asked.

"Well, you know how you paint up a horse's legs at the track to sweat a tendon using DMSO?" I asked.

"Oh yeah, that stuff works good to bring down a bow, just stinks something terrible," Paul said.

"Well, we're gonna give her a pretty big dose IV," I said, opening up the IV line to the liter of Ringer's containing the DMSO.

"I heard about using it IV on the track," Paul said. "The horse is supposed to smell like bad fish, boiled cabbage, and garlic for days when you do."

Within minutes after beginning the IV DMSO, the filly's breath began to smell of everything that Paul had just mentioned. "Whew, Doc, she's beginning to stink some now," Paul commented.

"Yup, she's gonna leave a vapor trail behind her for the next few days," I confirmed.

If there was ever a silver bullet for treating cerebral hypoxia, inflammation, and edema in horses, the IV administration of dimethyl sulfoxide (DMSO) would be it. It's also the bad-smelling stuff that you would likely have applied to the back of a horse's leg to reduce the inflammation associated with a tendinitis or a splint, and it's at the top of the list of ingredients on any number of emollients and salves used on the track as a sweat or blister.

DMSO is cheap, effective, smells awful, and has the unique property of swiftly crossing epithelial membranes. The ability of DMSO to migrate quickly across epithelial barriers has everything to do with why it works so well. It rapidly crosses skin, which is an epithelial membrane, and also the epithelial lining of blood vessels to reach the nervous system.

When a horse comes barreling out the back end of a trailer, flips over, and sustains a head injury, DMSO is the powerful anti–inflammatory that's given IV to reduce the water on the brain, or cerebral edema, that's likely to ensue from the fall. It also has the capability to increase cerebral blood flow, which of course means more oxygen to injured neurons.

I lubed up one end of a foal-size stomach tube and slid it up her nostril, down her esophagus, and into her stomach. "We're almost ready to get some groceries to her. Let's just tape the other end of this tube to her halter and get some milk from the mare," I said.

"Is the mare pretty good about milking her out?" I asked Paul.

"Yeah, she's easy, Doc, she doesn't care. She's got milk

like a cow and just 'bout lifts her leg when you go to milk her," Paul answered.

"This will be easier and safer than trying to bottle-feed her" I said to Paul. "She can get six to eight ounces of milk every hour through the tube until she can nurse on her own."

"Easy, Doc," Paul replied.

I went over to the mare, knelt down by her udder, and milked out a pint or so of milk into a plastic container. "You're right, Paul, she milks out like a Holstein cow," I commented. I filled up a dose syringe and gave the filly eight ounces of milk through the feeding tube.

"It's gonna be a bit of work but you'll need to get eight ounces of milk to her every hour for the next couple of days," I said to Paul.

"We got lots of help, Doc, won't be a problem, and besides, giving her milk through that tube will be faster than trying to bottle-feed her," Paul replied.

The ability to suck and swallow seems so automatic, so effortless, and so reflexive. We do it from a straw without even thinking. And yet the coordinated activity of dozens of paired muscle groups, the spinal cord, brain stem, and at least six of the twelve paired cranial nerves are all simultaneously involved.

As we watch in wonder a newborn foal nursing for the first time, we likely don't appreciate the neural feats of wizardry involved in the flow of life-giving milk from the mare's udder to the foal's stomach. A newborn foal, however, that has sustained cerebral injury at the time of birth struggles to do what seems so basic and so reflexive. Like an electrical outage that results in a partial blackout, the neural circuitry of that part of the nervous system that controls everything reflexive and automatic, including the ability to swallow, has been compromised.

The autonomic nervous system is the part of our nervous system that does everything automatic. It orchestrates almost all the responses we don't have to think about, and even though it's pretty much backstage, its functions are critical in getting us through the day.

Imagine what life would be like if we had to consciously manage the intricacies of digestion, heart rate, temperature regulation, blood pressure, and trying to remember to breathe while sleeping.

What if during a camping trip you were suddenly chased by a bear? As you frantically look how best to escape, would you remember the correct number of micrograms of adrenaline your adrenal glands need to secrete to help you run faster, or might you be off by a decimal point?

Would you remember to dilate your airways and constrict your peripheral circulation so that more blood could be diverted to your heart and lungs, helping you make your getaway? And what if, after your narrow escape, you were describing your adventure with friends over a meal. The responsibility of having to consciously manage the necessary timed release of your pancreatic enzymes during the telling of the tale would likely be somewhat of a distraction.

"She's gonna keep you guys busy over the next couple of days and I'll write everything down that she's going to need to have done," I said to Paul, taking out a notepad.

"Not a problem, Doc. Like I told ya, we got lots of help."

Tube feeding the filly hourly seems as if it should mimic the frequency with which a healthy foal would nurse on its own but actually, between lots of catnaps, a healthy foal will nurse an average of seven times in an hour. Over the course of the day this tallies out to about three to four gallons of milk, which means that a mare with a foal by her side produces over twelve hundred pounds of milk per month.

"Paul, if you finish giving her the plasma I'll check the mare's placenta."

"Sure thing, Doc. It's in a bucket outside the stall."

"Toxic shock" is frequently the outcome of a mare retaining any portion of her placenta. A type of uterine infection termed endometritis develops within only a matter of hours. Bacterial toxins result in the mare spiking a fever, colicking, and developing an often life-ending acute severe lameness known as "foal founder."

I laid the fifteen-pound-or-so placenta out on the floor of the barn aisle and examined both surfaces of each of the two distinct placental sacs. The smoky-gray amnionic sac was normal in color, texture, and appearance, as was the allantoic sac.

"It looks good," I called out to Paul. "It's all here and nothing to suggest that anything was wrong with the pregnancy that might have caused the problem last night with the filly coming out wrong."

I left instructions and an assortment of medications that the filly would need over the next few days, including another couple of doses of IV DMSO. I had treated several maladjusted foals in the past and some had turned the corner, but unfortunately others had not. It was a roll of the dice and time would tell.

It had been a bit of a long morning with Gipsy Maid's filly. I had taken blood from the filly to run some tests and would call Paul the next day with the results.

I drove out the eucalyptus-lined dirt road across the

bridge and pulled off the road a mile or so down Highway 1. It had become somewhat of a routine as I headed home, one that seemed to help return a bit of perspective and balance to my life. I walked along a favorite coastal bluff, a windswept promontory overlooking the rocky headlands below that jutted out into the Pacific. It was spring and the poppies, lupines, and irises were in bloom. The bluff was precipitous, steep-sided, and below was a favorite haul-out site for seals that gathered and packed together on the rocks. I sat down and smiled watching the seals below basking in the sun. A brown pelican was about to make a splash in the ocean. It had folded its wings from aloft and begun a plunge dive after sighting the reflected sunlight off the silvery scales of schooling fish below.

I THOUGHT ABOUT MY DAD and my last few days with him. I was in college at the time in Ohio and had received a message that he didn't have much more time. I had seen him last when I was eight years old and it had been fifteen years since. He had developed a rare form of cancer at age forty-eight and returned to California after living in the Philippines for many years. He wanted to spend what little time he had left in the Buttermilks along the eastern foothills of the Sierra Nevada, returning to die in the place where he had grown up.

The collage of emotions I experienced surrounding the death of my father was a spectrum of sorts—spectral in the way that as light passes through a prism it is divided, varied, with overlapping edges having the colors of the rainbow but with extremes at both ends.

Because so many years had passed since I had seen him, I felt I was on my way to say good-bye to someone I had never met. In another sense, however, his presence in my life as a child and even his later absence was the impetus that set in motion my own journey of exploration and discovery.

Paradox surrounded so much of what I felt at the time of his death. He had been at once both absent and present in my life, and as he waited to see me after so many years, he was in a sense holding on so he could let go. There would be joy in seeing him after so many years and yet sadness in seeing him leave once again.

The few days at the end of his life would be a distillation of sorts for both of us. I sought resolution, love, and understanding. He sought forgiveness and the hope that a part of him would always remain in my life.

It was his last day and I was all the family that was there as he slipped in and out of consciousness. I reminisced about the wonderful years in Jamaica. He listened and I thought I saw him smile as I remembered flying above the clouds, buying sugarcane juice with ice from the street vendors in Kingston, and holding each other's hands under water as the ocean waves passed above us at Treasure Beach.

IT WAS LATE IN THE MORNING ON THE FOURTH DAY after the filly had been born and Paul had left an all-too-brief message on my cell phone, wanting to know if I could come out to the farm that afternoon.

I felt a bit uneasy as I crossed the bridge, turned down the eucalyptus- and coastal pine–lined dirt road, and parked outside the broodmare barn. I hadn't returned Paul's message, sensing that perhaps the filly had taken a turn for the worse and that Paul had made the decision that the time had come to put her down.

I often tell clients somewhat facetiously that horses

should all be born with big red-and-white FRAGILE stickers. They're delicate, they break easy, and buying them is the cheapest part about owning them: It's fixing them that gets expensive.

"What was I thinking?" I wondered when I saw Paul standing outside the barn. This whole thing with the filly had been a lot of work and perhaps a bit more than just a hopeful stretch on my part. I had offered Paul a false sense of hope, the outcome of which after the investment of time, energy, and expense would be disappointment.

I opened the door to my truck and turned off the engine. "Hey, Doc, thanks for coming by," Paul said.

"Not a problem, and in fact I was meaning to give you a call to check on the filly," I replied, anticipating the news that I sensed was about to follow.

As we headed into the barn, I turned down the aisle toward Gipsy Maid's stall. "Wrong way, Doc, she ain't there no more," Paul said as he kept on walking.

"What happened?" I asked.

"This way, Doc, I'll show you," Paul replied. We headed out the other end of the barn to go back outside.

"It's been going on all morning long," Paul said grinning as we stood outside one of the turnout paddocks, and I stood and watched in near disbelief. "The mare's breaking a sweat trying to keep up with her," Paul added.

There was Gipsy Maid, galloping down the long side of the paddock trying to keep up with her filly, who was an easy couple of lengths in front of her like she was off to the races.

"She's been nursing good on her own since yesterday, Doc, so I pulled the catheter and stomach tube. Come this morning she's in the stall running around wanting to buck and play so I figured I'd turn 'em both out," Paul said. "It's like you said the other day, Doc."

"What do you mean?" I asked.

"Ya know, that thing you said about the filly that just because she's slow coming out of the starting gate doesn't mean she can't win the race."

{FOURTEEN}

City of Joy

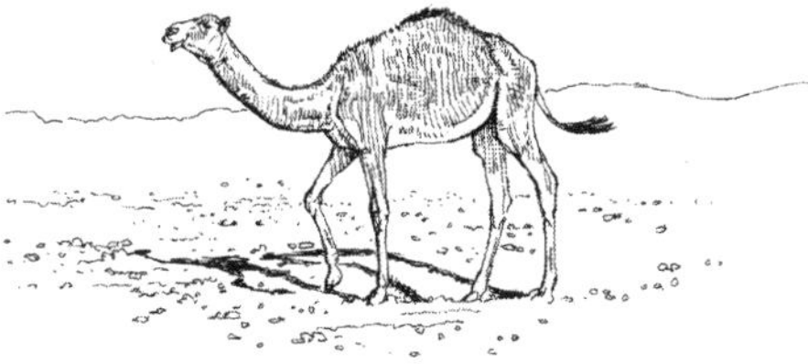

I ARRIVED IN THE CAPITAL PORT CITY of the Indian state of West Bengal during monsoon season. It was my nineteenth birthday. What little I owned was in a rucksack. I was young, alone, and amidst the chaotic sprawl of fourteen million people, most of whom were slum dwellers at a time when India was at its most broken and poor. My brief two-month visit coincided with a time when the Bangladesh Liberation War had led to a sea of ten million refugees pouring into East India, most of them arriving in Calcutta. British Crown rule of India had ended in 1947. Among the billion or so people in India, over four hundred different languages are spoken. Hindi and English predominate but confusion prevails. I didn't speak any Hindi or Bengali and *City of Joy*, a novel about the slums of Calcutta, was yet to be written.

My time in India wasn't intended to be a vision quest or a rite of passage, but as I look back I suppose in some ways that's what it was. After all, a journey is essentially a discovery of sorts, whether about a place or oneself.

I had heard about Mother Teresa's work in Calcutta but I was at an age where I was both naïve and ignorant. Her Missionaries of Charity were at best the subject of fleetingly glanced-at news items having little if any significance in my own life.

As I walked the slums in Calcutta, however, I saw some of her near countless homes for the homeless, the orphans, the lepers, and the dying in places such as abandoned Hindu temples. Noble and heroic was her mission to allow people who had "lived like an animal in the street . . . to die like an angel, loved and cared for."

Spiritual growth often begins from a place of turmoil and struggle. Developing a sense of compassion or the ability to *see the pain and feel the same* doesn't require spending time with the bereft and destitute in a place like India, but it helps.

Despite the crush of the populace in India, my time there would be spent very much alone. It would be a place of beginnings for me and an awakening of sorts. The realization that there was more to life would begin in a place of very much less.

My first chai spiced milk tea cost less than three cents. A dried cow-dung patty was the source of fuel to boil the water, and the milk that was added was from a water buffalo. I picked out the flecks and paid the few rupees.

My mother's book *Manners for Young People*, which she coauthored with my dancing school instructor in New York, didn't mention the customary usage of eating with one's right hand and wiping with one's left. Emily Post's book *Etiquette* doesn't reference it either, and yet that's what most of the world does. In places like India, where most people cannot afford the cost of firewood to cremate their dead, the hygienic practice of right and left has to do with the fact that toilet paper is an extravagance.

I lived on less than three dollars a day in India. It required my being somewhat resourceful but not really—after all, I was living on double what most Indians made in a day. I looked forward to my daily shower in the monsoon rains that came in daily from the Bay of Bengal. The horrific stench in the public bathrooms became less bothersome and using the stand over a hole in the floor where one squats was just that.

The meat and fish markets in Calcutta, Delhi, and Bombay were all similar. The slaughterhouse was also the marketplace. It was everything chaotic and macabre. There were rows of headless goats for sale lying in pools of blood, cleaver-waving butchers chasing off the crows perched on the hind quarters of recently butchered carcasses, and dogs everywhere licking up the spilled blood. Refrigeration was and still is nonexistent in most fish and meat markets in India. The meat one bought was still warm, often still twitching and from an animal slaughtered as one waited in line.

Calcutta is a port city, so a lot of Bengalese food is about fish. *Macher jhol* is a watery fish curry I bought from the street vendors. Salted lassi—buffalo-milk yogurt spiced with cumin—was what I sometimes had for dessert. And I ate a lot of mangoes. Unlike the privileged women in their saris who would flaunt their midriff rolls of fat like a Gucci handbag or a pair of Prada sunglasses, a status symbol showing that they were not one of the impoverished, I would lose twenty pounds.

Budget backpacker hostels were mainstream in Europe

but not so easy to find in places like Calcutta when I was there. From the fifty or so dollars a week I made over the previous year in Australia, I had saved some money but not a lot. I bought a one-way open plane ticket with flexible stopovers back to the States and would have to budget the rest.

As a result, I stayed in rooms with sheet-covered straw beds, in the stifling summer heat and humidity of India. The cockroaches were attracted to my sweat at night and I would sweep them off my chest.

It was odd to think that no one knew where I was. My dad, I would later find out, had moved to the island of Mindanao in the Philippines. My sister at age fifteen had run away to England and would eventually come to live in Dharamsala, a city in northern India, for twelve years. My mother was struggling in New York City. She was experiencing a series of nervous breakdowns that would require hospitalization.

I took a lot of buses and trains when I left Calcutta and headed a thousand miles south to Madras (now renamed Chennai), the capital city of Tamil Nadu. The ranch manager in Australia had given me the contact information of a couple of friends of his in India. One was a coffee plantation owner in the south of India outside the city of Mysore and the other was a sheep farmer north of Delhi. I would visit them both.

"Bustling" sounds somehow civilized and not at all descriptive of the Indian railways at that time. "Chaos," "havoc," and "pandemonium" are much more appropriate. The word "locomotive" must have its roots in India because "crazy" is everything about Indian train travel.

I took train rides where there were seemingly as many

people hanging on to the outside of the train as there were inside. The seats, aisles, and floors were always a crush of people, but fortunately there was usually extra seating available on the roof. It was both scenic and breezy, and I would join the hundreds already there.

My few days at the coffee plantation outside Mysore included a shower. I was in the mountainous south of India where it was cool and green. Working elephants moved timber and water buffalo plowed the fields. I learned how coffee is grown and I chatted with the respected and admired mahouts, the keepers of the working elephants.

A young boy will grow up with a baby elephant and together they will develop a lifetime relationship of trust and affection. The elephants respond with great loyalty and come to obey their mahout's voice and touch.

I WAS ON A TRAIN TO AGRA TO SEE THE TAJ MAHAL and then on to the desert state of Rajasthan in northern India. The landscape was changing and so was the wildlife. Instead of the free-roaming cows that add to an already chaotic traffic situation in the streets of Calcutta, the scavenging and dangling rhesus macaque monkeys were seemingly everywhere, climbing free in the train stations, temples, and streets of Delhi.

I had taken a rickety bus for a couple of hours from Jaipur to a small desert village where the Australian government had set up an experimental project in Rajasthan to study the viability of sheep farming in that part of India.

It was August and the desert heat was almost unbearable. As I walked along the road, I could see a dust storm approaching and was gestured to seek shelter in a nearby enclosure with others.

It happened to be a caravanserai, a walled but open-sky courtyard in the middle of which were hundreds of camels. It was a stopover of sorts, a not too uncommon type of place in northern India where camels rest up and are fed and watered.

A mobile camel clinic had been set up near the center of the courtyard, and I watched an Indian veterinarian treat a camel for a hump injury, while another camel waiting to be seen was holding its foot up.

Camels are seemingly everywhere in northern India, pulling carts loaded with kindling, logs, and sacks of feed. They're tons tougher than horses and can pull a heavier cart than an ox. They are even used to deliver the mail to many of the remote villages.

There were also small shops in the courtyard selling food, clothes, and other supplies. They also had a "Drome-dairy," a tented shop where for a few rupees you could buy a bowl of camel milk. Ice is not to be found in the remote villages of Rajasthan, so camel milk is usually served up warm and fresh, usually in a bowl. It's salty tasting. Water is sparse in that part of India, so when you hand the bowl back it's rinsed and swished with only a small bit of water and passed to the next customer.

I arrived at the sheep farm but spent the next few days in bed. There were monkeys in the trees outside my window. I was feverish, in a near constant sweat with abdominal cramps and diarrhea. The Australian I was staying with asked me if I saw blood in my diarrhea, and after I told him I had, he went to the village dispensary and brought me back some antibiotics.

Sheep's milk yogurt and mangoes were what I ate until I was strong enough to return to Jaipur to take a train to Bombay.

"SPIRITUAL" AND "MYSTICAL" were not words I used much when I was nineteen, nor would they have described my brief couple of months in India. My time of travel in the cities and remote villages of India didn't lead to a destination of "enlightenment" or "transcendent knowing," lofty words that appeared on tracts handed to me on the subways of New York by orange-robed Hare Krishnas. A profound shift in consciousness was not what I felt I had experienced as I left Bombay having lost twenty pounds and thinking that perhaps I had dysentery.

My experience in India, however, was the beginning of the realization that more could be found in less, an appreciation for what I did have rather than what I didn't. The insightful spiritual admonishment to spend more time looking at the donut rather than the hole is likely not to be referenced in any philosophical treatise on the Eastern religions, but in doing so I found my perception of life changed.

{FIFTEEN}

The Healing Power of Horses

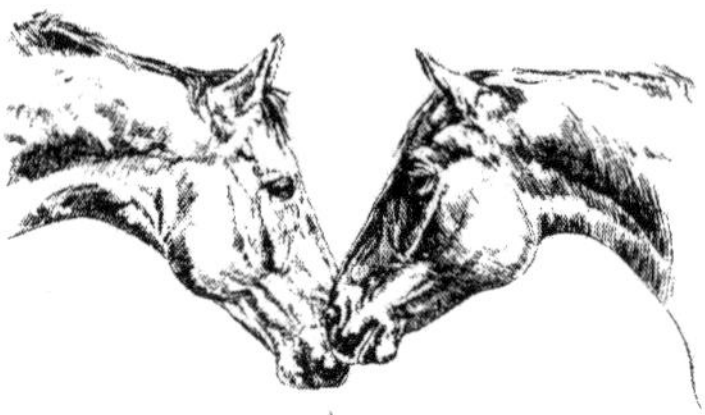

I PULLED UP IN FRONT OF THE STABLE at Pegasus Farm to check on Belle, one of their horses that had injured her eye. Sally, the barn manager, had left a message on my cell phone earlier in the day asking me to come out as soon as possible. I had been doing their work for quite some time and Sally knew, as I did, that eye injuries are always an emergency.

Belle was a big girl and she had an important job. She was a twenty-two-hundred-pound, chestnut-colored Belgian mare and was one of the sixteen or so therapeutic riding horses at Pegasus Farm.

The Belgian breed of draft horse, as the name implies, is native to Belgium. This little country is blessed with fertile soil and abundant rainfall, providing the farmers of Belgium with the excellent pastures, hay, and grain necessary to develop a heavy, powerful, and very kind breed of horse.

Belle was certainly just that, as sweet as she was big, and anyone who had spent any time around horses would have described her as an "easy keeper." It didn't take much in the way of groceries for her to put the weight on, and although she was heavier than she should have been I could never quite bring myself to think of her as being overweight. "Well nourished" seemed a kinder way of describing her plus-size when it came to her girth, shoes, and bridle.

I had been out of veterinary school for many years before I became familiar with the term or concept of a therapeutic riding horse. Of course, I knew that riding a horse was therapeutic, but in a broader and more casual context of the word, more perhaps in the recreational sense of being therapeutic, and not curative by any means.

"Alternative therapeutic modalities" as a strategy in approaching a disease or disorder had not yet been integrated into the medical curricula when I was a veterinary student.

My veterinary medical training had been traditional rather than "alternative," and acupuncture, herbal supplements, and chiropractic manipulations of the horse were never mentioned. My impression of the word "alternative" at the time had more to do with a California lifestyle than an approach to medicine.

My concept of something being therapeutic meant that it was to be found in a pill bottle, a medicated powder, or a vial of injectable medication. I was taught that healing was to be imparted by a medicinal substance found on a pharmacy shelf and therapy was something you went through while lying on a couch. I was old school and obviously had no idea at the time how the world of both human and veterinary medicine would soon change.

It's unlikely that doctors in the past would have scribbled out for their ailing patients a prescription that included whinnies and nickers. Therapeutic protocols described in medical textbooks years ago would have offered up electroshock therapy rather than a trip to the barn for any number of neuromuscular disorders and emotional disabilities.

The notion that horses could in a very real way be therapeutic was an astonishing revelation for me. Pegasus Farm would be my introduction to a truly remarkable dimension of medicine I didn't know existed.

If I was there for routine immunizations or to attend to an injured horse, I would always find some time afterwards to wander down to the riding ring and watch as the magic unfolded.

Belle saw several patients a day, including a young boy by the name of Brian.

Brian was an eight-year-old boy who had a developmental disorder characterized by emotional detachment and impaired communication. He was like many autistic children in that he seldom smiled. His social skills were clearly limited, and he appeared to live in a world of his own. He was a recluse of sorts, unwilling to look you in the eye, emotionally distant, and seemingly almost fearful and wounded. He wasn't obviously physically challenged, and yet it was clear that he seemed somehow rigid, unable to relax, and that he struggled with coordination.

As Brian was led up to the mounting block, things were about to change: Belle would work her magic.

Belle was ever so patient as she stood at the mounting block while three people helped Brian saddle up. One person would stand at the front of Belle holding her halter, with another person on either side to steady Brian once he swung his leg over the saddle.

"Why is therapeutic riding so therapeutic?" I asked the

Ph.D. physical therapist who was standing next to me one day as we both watched Brian, sitting atop Belle, being led around the ring.

"All of a sudden, their world changes," he said. "The child's brain is dazzled by the smell, the feel, the touch, the rhythmical walk, the sound of a nicker, and the warmth of the horse's body. Sluggish and distant neurons in remote parts of Brian's brain begin to light up like a pinball machine."

"You're kidding," I exclaimed.

"Absolutely not," he emphasized.

He described how the child's body would quickly fall into sync with the rhythmical walk of the horse. "It's like a dance," he said. "The child will follow the horse's lead. The horse swings its hips as it walks and the child mimics the motion. It sounds a bit Zen, but the horse teaches the kid to relax, something most of them don't know how to do."

As I watched, I could see it begin to happen. Brian's motion was becoming Belle's motion. His rigidity and tension seemed to fade with each footfall of Belle's.

In Ph.D. lingo, the therapist went on to explain how not only would Brian's cognition improve with time in the saddle but his speech as well. "Brian's perception of the world changes in a wonderful way when he sits in the saddle. It's pretty empowering stuff when these kids are suddenly ten feet tall and no longer feeling as helpless as they do most of the time," the therapist commented.

"Have a look. Can you see what's happening now? Brian is starting to give a smile, kind of a rare thing to see with these kids, and the horses make it happen."

My concept of what was therapeutic was changing with the realization that the impaired ability of a child to think, speak, and perform complex motor skills could be remedied by something that eats hay and lives in a barn.

The boundaries of medicine were also changing—shifting and expanding as those involved in the health care professions were discovering that what is healing and medicinal is not limited to the confines of a pill bottle.

"I THINK SHE'S GOT SOMETHING IN THERE but she won't let me open her eye to have a look," Sally said as we headed into the barn.

I went into Belle's stall and could see that her right eye was almost closed. She was squinting and tearing from the pain, and as I gently tried to pry open her eyelids, she squeezed her eye shut.

"I'll be right back. I need to grab some gear from the truck," I said to Sally.

"All right, Sally, let's see if we can get a better look," I said when I returned with my ophthalmic kit. I drew up some medication into a syringe and attached a small-gauge pediatric needle. "Okay, Sally, here we go. Hang on to her halter and steady her head while I give her this injection."

The injection I was about to give wasn't one that is given into a vein or the muscle; instead it was given around a nerve, and almost anybody who has been to the dentist has had one. It's called a nerve block and it's achieved by giving a "local."

There are lots of different types of local anesthetics that physicians, dentists, and veterinarians use. Some are stronger than others, some last longer, and others are rapid in onset (these fast-acting ones are those most preferred by dental patients).

Novocain, the local anesthetic that dental patients and

others are most familiar with, is actually the trade name for procaine. There is also lidocaine, bupivacaine, mepivacaine, proparacaine, and many, many more. They all seem to end in "–aine," which rhymes with what they're supposed to do: block the pain.

Most people are aware that a local anesthetic is given before a cavity is drilled or a wound is stitched. But many people don't realize that a local anesthetic can also be used to block the nerve that allows a muscle to function. This is why, after you have been given a local for a cavity filling, not only can you not feel that area of your gum, but often your lip is droopy as well. The embarrassment of having your friend tell you that you are drooling is understandably explained away when you reveal you have just seen the dentist.

Horses are not so keen on instruments and hands approaching their eyes, so what do they do? They squeeze their eyelids shut. It's the predictable response by almost all horses when an attempt is made to do an eye exam.

The fact that a muscle needs a nerve to function is a bit of neurophysiology taken advantage of when a veterinarian reaches for a vial of local anesthetic.

"That should take just a minute to kick in, Sally, and then we'll be able to have a look," I said after injecting a bit of mepivacaine around Belle's auriculopalpebral nerve—a small nerve a couple of inches above her right eye that provided motor function to the *orbicularis oculi*, the blink muscle of Belle's right eye.

It's an odd way to spend a thought but think what would happen if we couldn't blink. The muscles around our eyes that allow us to blink are vital, even though they're likely not the ones that men try and flex when standing in front of a mirror. If we didn't have blink muscles, our eyelids would not be able to function as the windshield wipers of our eyes. Being able to blink is somewhat similar to what happens when the big-rig semi blows by our car on a rainy day on the freeway, leaving our windshield covered in road spray and truck splash. We have trouble seeing until we flip the windshield wipers on.

"That worked pretty fast," Sally said as I turned the light of my ophthalmoscope on.

"Yup, that little local works well. Sort of makes their muscle go dishrag flaccid pretty quick. Have a feel now of her eyelid," I said to Sally.

"Wow, she can't squeeze her eye shut, and her eyelid feels like it has gone limp," Sally remarked as she lifted Belle's eyelid this way and that. "Her eye is all red. What'd she do?" Sally asked.

"I'm not sure, but let's have a closer look," I said.

I numbed up Belle's cornea, the glassy surface of her eye, with a couple of drops of another type of local so she wouldn't feel what would happen next. "Sally, I need your help. Hang on to my ophthalmoscope and shine the light in her eye when I tell you." I took out a six-inch cotton swab. "Okay, let's go," I said, holding up Belle's eyelid with one hand and using the cotton swab in my other to sweep high up under her eyelid.

"Here's the problem, Sally, have a look," I said, showing her what was on the end of the cotton swab. "It was hiding up in the conjunctival sac under her eyelid.".

"What is it?" she asked.

"It's a grass awn, a little torpedo-shaped seed covered with barbs. No wonder her eye was so red. It must have blown into her eye while she was eating her hay or out grazing.

"We need to see if she scratched her cornea," I added, taking out a fluorescein dye strip and gently placing it on the surface of her eye.

"What's that gonna do?" Sally asked.

"If that grass awn abraded her eye, the dye will turn green and fluoresce where she scratched her cornea," I explained.

When I shone my ophthalmoscope on her eye, I saw the neon-green staining, paintbrush-like streak marks across more than 60 percent of her cornea. "Have a look, Sally. She got a pretty good rub on her cornea," I said.

"Wow, no wonder she had her eye closed, it must have been awfully painful," Sally remarked.

"I bet she made matters worse, however."

"Why? What do you mean?" Sally asked.

"Did you see her rubbing her face on her leg?" I asked.

"That's exactly what she was doing before you came," Sally answered.

Horses are just like people in that when they get something in their eye, the itchy sensation that follows makes them want to rub the eye. Horses obviously don't have fingers, so instead they rub their faces up and down their legs. The effect is the same: Rubbing an itchy eye that has a foreign body typically results in more trauma to the delicate cornea.

I explained to Sally that despite the paintbrush-like abrasions affecting most of her cornea, Belle was actually somewhat fortunate in that the lesions were superficial. The cornea would heal within three to four days. Sally would need to administer some ophthalmic ointment several times per day to the affected eye, as well as give Belle some Banamine paste, an oral anti-inflammatory medication used in horses.

After showing Sally how to administer the ointment into Belle's eye, I explained that the affected eye should appear much more comfortable over the next few days. "The squinting and tearing should begin to subside within a day, and she can go back to work tomorrow," I said. "Of course, give me a call if it hasn't," I added.

I handed Sally a couple of tubes of eye ointment and headed out of the barn toward my truck. Then I turned back. "Hey, Sally, I think I'll swing by in a few days and have a look at her just to be sure. Not to worry, there won't be a charge," I smiled.

I knew that Belle would be fine when I came back to check on her in a few days. I would of course have a look at her and make sure she was on the mend, but I would also wander down to the ring and see more of the magic unfold.

{SIXTEEN}

Colic 101: The Inside Story

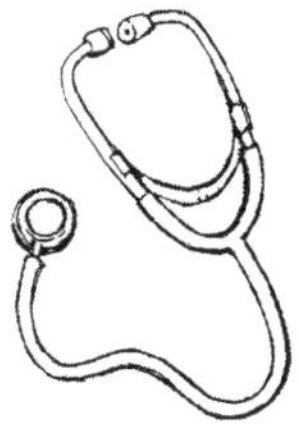

"ACUTE ABDOMEN OF UNKNOWN ETIOLOGY." This is what the ER physician would scribble on his intake notes if you were to walk into the emergency room complaining of the sudden onset of abdominal cramps.

The ER doc examining you has no idea of course whether your stomachache is from the bad sushi you ate last night, or perhaps from an appendicitis in the works, or possibly the result of a section of gas-distended bowel.

"Acute onset colic" is what a horse vet would enter in their medical records after examining a colicky horse in the barn. The etiology—or cause—of abdominal pain in horses is just as wide-ranging as the cause of abdominal pain in humans.

From literally hundreds of different etiologies that can result in an "acute abdomen," how does the ER doc begin to sort out what is the cause behind your particular abdominal pain? Food poisoning may resolve with a bit of "tincture of time," whereas an about-to-burst appendix requires you to hop aboard a fast-moving gurney to the operating room.

A veterinarian examining a colicky horse in the barn late at night is similarly wondering, Why is the horse colicking? Is it something the horse ate, perhaps a bit of moldy hay or grain? Is there an underlying tumor or abdominal abscess? Is it a gas colic, a spasmodic colic, or perhaps a twisted gut? Is it a simple constipation or a complicated torsion of the large intestine that will require immediate surgery? Any number of etiologies are possible as to what might be responsible for the abdominal pain, including stress ulcers.

The world of human medicine has only in recent years come to realize how profoundly the phenomena of stress affects our health. Pharmaceutical companies have responded by developing anti–ulcer medications such as Nexium and Prilosec to treat such disorders as esophagitis, gastric ulcers, and inflammatory bowel disease.

Veterinarians have also come to realize more fully just how much stress factors into an array of abdominal disorders in horses. Medications such as GastroGard (omeprazole), Zantac (ranitidine), Tagamet (cimetidine), and Carafate (sucralfate) are all anti-ulcer medications now available to treat stress-related bowel disease in horses. An assortment of over-the-counter anti-ulcer products is also available, including Pepto-Bismol, which by the way horse vets purchase by the gallon, and Neigh-Lox, the equine equivalent of the antacid for people, Maalox.

It seems odd that the intangible phenomenon of stress is a significant causal factor of colic or abdominal pain in horses. Horse vets readily agree that stress is less of a distinct disease or syndrome, but rather more of a "nebulopathy," a vague and shadowy villain of sorts. The lingering backdrop of stress provides a stage or setting where other disorders are allowed to come into play.

You might be wondering, What could possibly be stressful for a horse? Actually, many causes of stress in horses are very similar to the stressors in our own lives. Major life changes, being too busy, not enough down time, rocky relationships at the barn, changes in weather, and especially a break in a horse's routine, are all very stressful. Financial pressures are considered a source of stress in our lives and perhaps that is also the case in a horse's life if it means an eventual shortage of hay and grain.

Horses are creatures of habit. Whether it's what they eat or when they are turned out, horses like a routine. Disrupting their daily routine by putting them on a trailer to ship to a show out of state where they are stabled away from home for several nights can be enormously stressful.

The world of equine medicine has advanced tremendously over the last few years. Unfortunately, the "3 *B*'s" of Civil War equine medicine—bleeding, blistering, and burning—persisted well into the twentieth century. Attempts to heal sick and injured horses were archaic and at times more cruel than they were remedying.

The United States lagged behind Europe in supporting the development of veterinary schools. In fact, America would not have its first veterinary school until the 1850s. Eurasia had for centuries relied upon the horse, whether ridden or driven, in times of both war and peace. Crucial in battle, essential in agriculture, and vital to transport, the horse was a foundation of the success of European nations for hundreds of years. Medical care and knowledge of the horse in Europe evolved from the understanding that the health of a nation was critically coupled to the health of its horses and livestock.

The Civil War would bring about the formation of dozens of cavalry regiments in both the Union and Confederate armies requiring the service of thousands of horses. And yet, as late as 1863, there were only six veterinarians in the Union army. In that same year, the Union army would lose seventeen thousand horses to "glanders," a highly contagious respiratory disease of horses caused by the bacterium *Pseudomonas mallei*. As with the soldiers, the large concentration of horses in close proximity to each other provided a fertile ground for any number of infectious diseases.

Giant horse infirmaries were set up by both Union and Confederate cavalries during the Civil War, an early impetus for the advance of veterinary medicine. Tragically, however, little was understood about diseases of horses and their transmission. Nonetheless, this would be a pivotal time in the world of veterinary medicine as the United States government would soon initiate funding for the formation of veterinary medical schools.

The advance of equine medicine would still be slow in coming. Not all that many years ago, a bullet between the ears was all that was left to do with a horse with a fractured leg. Industrial solvents, dry cleaning agents, and toxic organophosphates were administered to horses to treat any number of parasitic disorders. Turpentine was given to treat a horse with a bellyache, and arsenic was the drug of choice on the racetrack to give a horse's coat a better shine.

Equine sports physiology has only fairly recently abandoned much of what was once considered therapeutic in the treatment of equine athletic injuries. For far too many years the inflamed and torn tendons of horses were treated using the cruel and primitive practice of pin firing and blistering.

Dousing the tendon-inflamed legs of horses with caustic chemicals was done in hopes of "tightening up" tendons. "Counter-irritation" was the therapeutic strategy that justified taking multiple red-hot irons to "pin fire" the leg of a horse in hopes of treating a tendinitis.

The burning and blistering of the horse's leg would result in the skin becoming indurated and leather-like, all of which was somehow thought to facilitate healing. Outlawed in Europe yet still allowed in the United States, it would be analogous to treating your strained Achilles tendon with a soldering gun.

Antiquated in their use, blistering compounds are still to be found trackside and are applied to horses' legs to treat "sore" tendons. The mercurial-based solvents result in a chemical skin peel, leaving the horse's leg oozing and weeping serum, with the hopeful but skewed intent of improved healing after having done so.

Bloodletting was the treatment of choice not all that many years ago for horses suffering from laminitis. If drilling their feet somehow didn't allow enough blood to spill to the outside, jugular veins were incised in a 1–2-gallon bloodletting endeavor to facilitate the cure of the foundering horse.

Fortunately, equine sports medicine and therapeutics has greatly changed. Therapeutic protocols for equine injuries and ailments now parallel much of what takes place in human medicine.

Let's jump back to the ER room for a moment. The ER doc, just like the horse vet, knows that "a history well taken is a diagnosis half made" and so would like to ask you a few questions. Taking the time and insight to ask the right questions often reduces diagnostic efforts and hastens the arrival at an accurate diagnosis.

"What have you eaten recently?" If your answer includes raw oysters, old potato salad, or possibly undercooked hamburger, the physician would likely suspect that food poisoning is high on the list of possible etiologies. Food-borne pathogens seem to be on the rise, and bacteria like *Staphylococcus*, *E. coli*, and *Salmonella* are often the culprits.

"Do you have any pets?" he may ask. And in all likelihood you would wonder, Now why in the world would the ER doc find this information helpful? Knowing that snakes, turtles, lizards, and other reptiles are often a reservoir of infection for *Salmonella*, the sleuth-like skills of the physician are at work.

"Have you traveled outside the country recently?" If you answered yes, that indeed you had recently returned from Latin America, a tentative diagnosis of "tourista" would likely come to the forefront.

"Where exactly does it hurt?" If you responded that the pain seems to emanate particularly from your lower-right abdominal quadrant, the ER physician would be suspicious of an incipient appendicitis. If vomiting and fever accompanied the above symptoms, imminent rupture of your appendix would jump to the top of the list of likely diagnoses, and the OR would be called with a heads-up that you were on the way.

Further insightful inquiries made by the ER doc might help narrow down the list of possible etiologies and prevent you from having to endure the expense and effort of any number of unnecessary diagnostic medical procedures.

Similarly, the strategic questioning of the owner of the colicky horse in the barn by the veterinarian is equally of value in arriving at a correct diagnosis.

"Has there been any change in the horse's diet recently?"

"Has the horse recently returned from a show or competition?"

"Is he up-to-date on his vaccinations?"

"Has he ever colicked before?"

"Is the horse receiving any antibiotic or anti-inflammatory medication?"

"When was the horse last dewormed?"

While the veterinarian was assessing the color of the mucous membranes of the horse and taking its temperature, the list of questions would go on. "Is the horse a good water drinker? "Is he a good eater?" "Is he a cribber?" "Has he recently been exposed to any other sick horses?" Emphasizing once again that "a history well taken is a diagnosis half made," the Sherlock Holmes skills of a veterinarian can be both time- and lifesaving.

MY WIFE AND I WERE AWAKENED by the sound of our daughter crying loudly in her crib. I looked at the clock. It was almost 1:00 A.M. I jumped out of bed and knew as only a parent knows that these were not the cries that had gotten us out of bed in the past. These were the shrieks of pain.

My wife stayed at home with our other child as I made the midnight run to the emergency room of our community hospital. The shrill cries of pain continued for the duration of the half-hour trip to the hospital.

The ER doc asked me an array of questions while he poked and pressed on the little tummy of my daughter. She wasn't running a fever and there was no accompanying vomiting or diarrhea. The restraint and blood draw for a stat CBC (complete blood count) and chemistry panel was accompanied by an even louder shriek than those during the trip in.

It was after the abdominal radiographs were taken that I was called in to speak with the physician while the nurse took my daughter back to the exam room. “Voila, there’s the problem,” he said, pointing to one of the radiographs on the viewing screen. “Her large intestine is distended with gas and of course it’s quite painful.”

During our conversation, my daughter’s crying from the adjacent exam room suddenly stopped. A nurse then appeared with the good news that my daughter had passed some gas and the pain had subsequently subsided.

As I was about to leave the emergency room to head home with my daughter, the ER doc came up to me with some helpful advice. “I have seven kids of my own,” he said, “and what I am about to tell you won’t be found in any textbook on pediatric medicine. If this happens again, before you bring her in, sit her on the washing machine and turn it on spin cycle for ten minutes. If it’s a bit of trapped gas, that should fix her.”

Gas colic is not only a common cause of abdominal pain in infants, but is also frequently encountered in horses. Trapped gas causes distension of the affected piece of gut, resulting in the horse becoming painful. Horse vets will recommend a similar strategy to “spin cycle therapy” to jostle free the trapped gas. The horse is loaded on the trailer and taken down a bumpy road. If a trailer isn’t available, putting the horse on the lunge line for a few minutes at the trot will often free up the trapped gas pocket.

OF THE SEVENTY-FIVE TRILLION CELLS or so that make up the human body, billions and billions are nerve cells or neurons. Yes, of course a lot of neurons are in your brain, but a lot of them are also out there in your skin, muscles, and elsewhere, receiving and transmitting vital information.

One of the safety features that comes standard with your body is a remarkable warning system that alerts you to noxious stimuli. Unlike some of the crash avoidance features that cost extra on high-end luxury cars, this ingenious design feature provides an advanced warning system and comes standard on all horse and human models.

"Nociception" is the name of this detection and warning system, and nociceptors are the integral components that make it all happen.

Nociceptors are specialized neurons dedicated to detecting pain. These neurons are on the prowl and alert for "noxious stimuli," the medical term for that which is potentially injurious or harmful to your body. There are noxious fumes, noxious gases, noxious chemicals, and—I apologize, I couldn't help myself—obnoxious people.

Some nociceptor neurons detect things like thermal and chemical stimuli. Other nociceptors are "stretch receptor" neurons located in the wall of your intestine and elsewhere. They are capable of sending a volley of impulses through the sensory axon to your spinal cord, where they form several kinds of synapses resulting in the process of nociception—the perception of pain.

Stretch receptors light up when there is a mechanical distortion of our tissues. This is why you say "Ouch, that hurts!" when someone pinches your skin. Stretch receptors are also located in the wall of your intestine and transmit signals along the spinal cord to your brain, which results in the experience of pain when your gassy large bowel is beginning to balloon.

The neural process of encoding pain is essential to our survival, and the perception of pain is actually a good thing.

But wait, I sense that perhaps you are not so sure of that, and in fact I might initially agree.

Imagine how much more pleasant our lives would be if life was pain-free. Migraines wouldn't hurt, and we could laugh off the sting of a bee. You could rest your hand on the still-hot stove burner for as long as you liked, and our toe wouldn't hurt when stepped on by a horse. The finger caught in the car door would be of little consequence and the sprained ankle from a slip or fall would be but a fleeting concern.

On the other hand, if you didn't grimace and groan from the abdominal pain from your inflamed and about-to-burst appendicitis, you wouldn't have cause to go to the ER. Instead, your appendix would simply rupture, peritonitis and septicemia would rapidly ensue, and next of kin would be contacted.

The obstructed bowel of a horse with an impaction colic quickly begins to distend. The contents of the intestine—the ingesta—come to a sluggish standstill and, like a traffic jam on a busy interstate, the blockage prevents the passage of food down the pike. The stretch receptors in the wall of the horse's gut quickly begin to transmit pain signals to the horse's brain.

By the way, how does a colicky horse manifest pain? Most horse owners are familiar with the signs of colic in a horse, and very typically there's a progression of clinical signs that will occur as the pain becomes increasingly severe.

A horse with a mildly painful gut will simply go off its feed. Horse owners are well aware that horses don't eat to live but, rather, live to eat. When a horse isn't interested in its grain or hay, the owner begins to experience a worrisome concern.

If the abdominal pain progresses and becomes more severe, the horse will often be seen to turn to look at its belly, and on occasion may lift its lip in what's known as a flehmen response. Agitation ensues as the pain progresses and the horse may begin to seemingly pace the deck in its stall.

Increasing abdominal pain results in the horse's heart rate climbing and its blood pressure dropping. The horse is now becoming "shocky" and will often break into a sweat around its neck and shoulders. It will then begin to repeatedly paw, lie down, and roll. As the pain intensifies and becomes more and more relentless, the horse becomes uncontrollable and near violent.

Hopefully, long before the pain progresses to the point where the horse becomes uncontrollable, a veterinarian has been contacted to treat the animal. Fortunately, most colicky horses a veterinarian sees in the barn at night respond well to the treatment given, the outcome of which is a happy horse grazing in the paddock the next day. Early intervention is key.

If, however, veterinary medical intervention is not provided to the colicky horse, the cascade of events that follows is often tragic.

Regardless of whether or not the abdominal pain is a result of a strangulating twist, a displacement, or impaction, the endpoint leading to the horse's demise is the same: ischemic bowel.

Ischemia is the medical term used to describe a deficiency of arterial blood to tissues. Arterial blood, in contrast to venous blood, is the oxygen-rich side of the circulatory system. Arterial blood vessels are the lifelines of the circulatory system, bringing vital oxygen supplies to the intestinal wall and other tissues.

As arterial blood vessels are compressed by the affected bowel wall segment that is twisted or distended, inadequate tissue perfusion ensues. Diminishing oxygen supplies to the affected bowel wall activate those pain receptor neurons that detect changes in chemical stimuli. Plummeting tissue oxygen levels trigger neuron receptors to send additional pain signals to the horse's brain. The colicky horse becomes now even more painful.

The lack of oxygen in the ischemic bowel wall results in the devitalization of tissue. The capability of the intestinal wall to function as a protective barrier is compromised. Toxin-laden, lethal bacteria swiftly take advantage of the breach and begin their advance toward the horse's circulatory system.

If you were to peer inside the belly of the colicky horse at this point, what would you see? You would note that the color of the distended or twisted piece of gut wall has changed. It is no longer a healthy pink but has become more of a toxic brick red. Dwindling tissue oxygen will result in further devitalization of the bowel as it changes color once again to a cyanotic purple. "Necrosis" is the medical term for death of tissue, and black is the final color change of the now necrotic bowel.

The breach in the gut wall has allowed bacteria and their toxins access to the horse's bloodstream. The colicky horse will soon succumb to toxic shock.

Blood poisoning, septicemia, toxic shock, and septic shock are all synonymous terms for the way in which millions of people worldwide die in hospitals each year from endotoxemia.

Endotoxemia is the common death walk in people

suffering from pneumonia, pancreatitis, appendicitis, hepatitis, meningitis, pyelonephritis, and other infections.

Endotoxic shock is the number one cause of death in human hospital intensive care units. Similarly, endotoxic shock is why horses die from colic. Because the ischemic gut wall has lost its capability to function as a protective barrier, an inpouring of toxin-producing bacteria soon wreaks havoc with the horse's circulatory system.

The chaotic hematological events that subsequently occur in the circulatory system are both overwhelming and ultimately catastrophic.

But wait. In order to more clearly understand the end-stage physiological events surrounding endotoxic shock, a brief digression into the world of hematology may be helpful. Ready? Here we go.

Lunchtime is approaching and thoughts turn to an old favorite: soup and a sandwich. You take the can opener out of the drawer and because you are hungry and in a bit of a hurry, you somehow carelessly manage to slice your finger on the Campbell's Chicken Noodle Soup can lid.

After muttering an expletive or two, you head to the medicine cabinet to retrieve a Band-Aid and go back to making lunch. The cut on your finger is merely a bit of a nuisance in the scheme of things, and in all likelihood you don't give a passing thought to how your finger stopped bleeding, it just did.

Clotting factors and the "coagulation cascade" are not likely topics of your thought life unless you are perhaps a hematologist or are interested in the physiological events associated with toxic shock and the demise of a severely colicky horse.

How is it that your finger suddenly stopped bleeding

from the slice you sustained from the soup can lid while making yourself lunch?

The ability to clot bleeding blood simply seems like a given. We take enormously for granted the gifts of life, including the fact that we are born with the right clotting factors.

My high school classmate was incapable of producing the blood-clotting protein known as Factor VIII. He was a hemophiliac. What most of us consider minor nicks, scrapes, and bruises were life-threatening bleed-outs for him. Paper cuts and soup tin lid nicks were potential hemorrhagic events. For him, a bump on the head was a worrisome problem that could transition into an intracranial hemorrhage. The coroner's report would one day list "internal hemorrhage from a spontaneous bleeding episode" as the cause of his death, not long after his nineteenth birthday.

What if, instead of putting a Band-Aid on your cut finger, you put it under a microscope, magnifying life's events a thousand times. What would you see?

Peering through the microscope's lenses allows you to be visually transported down to the cellular level of life. As you bring the slice on your finger into focus, you would see the chaotic commotion of blood escaping from blood vessels and realize . . . you're bleeding!

Feeling somewhat queasy, you adjust the fine-focus knob to uncover further detail of the area of carnage. Preliminary damage assessment indicates substantial damage. As you survey the ragged ends of several severed blood vessels, your eyes widen, seeing the stuff of blood everywhere: blood cells of all sorts—red ones, white ones, and platelets—in a deluge of plasma. Collateral damage would include shredded epithelial skin cells and exposed and tattered connective tissue.

Staring in disbelief, you shake your head and

discouragingly conclude, "It doesn't look good." Epithelial skin cells have suffered heavy casualties, as have the endothelial cells that line the blood vessels. There is also widespread disruption of the surrounding collagenous matrix, and the hemorrhage seems to continue.

Hold on, what's that you see? Eagerly and enthusiastically you gaze at what seems to be a first response team beginning to muster. It's the platelets, and hundreds of thousands of them are rushing to the vascular break. Activated by having come in contact with the connective tissue stuff in your finger called collagen, they go into action.

"It's like a superhero Marvel comic," you think to yourself, watching the valiant and unified efforts of the platelets to stop the bleed. What are they doing now? you wonder as the platelets begin to change shape. Ordinarily spherical, they're becoming star-shaped and starting to grow pseudopods—literally "false feet." These pseudopodia are leglike projections that allow the platelets to more efficiently plug the leak in the damaged blood vessel.

"Yes, yes, yes!" you say, cheering the platelets on. "It's working! They're doing it!" you exclaim, seeing even more platelets arrive at the site of the severed blood vessel and join hands—or perhaps I should say pseudopodia—to create a platelet plug, or clot. Simultaneously, exposed collagen initiates the coagulation cascade, a series of enzymatic reactions that, within minutes, result in the formation of a fibrin protein fiber mesh. Another company of platelets arrives and reinforces the fibrin mesh clot. "They did it. They really did it," you hear yourself say: The bleeding has miraculously stopped.

You have every right to ask how any of this relates to the colicky horse that is about to succumb to endotoxic shock.

All of the above is merely an attempt to emphasize the fact that the coagulation cascade and the ability to clot blood are phenomena that enable us to stop bleeding. "Well, that seems fairly obvious," you might remark.

Okay, okay, here's my point and here's how all of this has a bearing on the colicky horse: Blood is supposed to clot in order to stop the bleeding or hemorrhage from a torn or damaged blood vessel. Blood is *not* supposed to clot when blood is *inside* a blood vessel.

"So what's the big deal if it does?" you ask. Good question.

If blood clots form inside our blood vessels, and on occasion they do, the medical literature has a plethora of terms to describe what follows, including the following: stroke, thrombus, embolus, infarction, heart attack, pulmonary embolism, and deep vein thrombosis . . . all not good.

A thrombus is the medical term to describe a blood clot in a blood vessel. If the thrombus breaks loose and floats downstream, it is then called an embolus. Thrombi and emboli block or occlude the supplying artery's ability to provide vital oxygen to the tissues downstream.

Infarction (not to be confused with the speeding ticket you are issued as a traffic "infraction") refers to tissue death caused by a lack of oxygen due to the obstruction of the tissue's blood supply.

Infarctions can occur in any tissue or organs. Regardless of whether the location is a lung, liver, spleen, or kidney, infarctions can be devastating. For example, an infarction in cardiac muscle would result from a thrombus in the heart's coronary artery, the oxygen-supplying artery to your heart. The occluding thrombus in your coronary artery stops the heart muscle tissue downstream receiving oxygen, and the oxygen-deprived muscle tissue subsequently necroses—it dies. This is called a myocardial infarction and is the way in which most heart attacks come about.

Similarly, a thrombus in one of the supplying arteries to your cerebrum—your brain—would result in a cerebral infarction, more commonly termed a "stroke."

Aspirin is an anticoagulant, and taking a baby aspirin once a day is generally a good thing. Aspirin is said to be a blood thinner, in other words it stops the blood from clotting in places where it's not supposed to, places like your coronary artery. Aspirin works to "thin out" the blood by inhibiting the activity of platelets: platelets are much less sticky when aspirin is around, much less apt to try and join up to form a clot.

There are lots of different anticoagulants used in hospitals, and even a few used in barns. Aspirin, heparin, and warfarin are frequently administered to hospital patients, and warfarin, the active ingredient in the rat and mouse poison d-Con, is used in barns.

Now, let's get back to the ischemic gut wall of the colicky horse. Lack of oxygen supply to that part of the horse's gut wall has resulted in tissue death. The devitalized section of bowel wall becomes a floodgate, a catastrophic breach allowing trillions of toxin-producing bacteria to make their advance toward the horse's circulatory system.

Most of the bacteria found in the horse's gut are wearing white hats, that is to say they're good guys. Both horse and bacteria not only coexist, but each mutually benefits from the other in a symbiotic relationship. The horse provides living accommodations for the bacteria, and in turn the bacteria aid with the digestion of the fibrous diet of the horse.

There are other bacterial organisms in the horse's gut,

however. These are the toxin-producing, gunslinging, black-hatted bad hombres, the gram-negative coliform types such as *E. coli* and *Pseudomonas.*

The lumen of the intestine is the space where the soupy mix of grain and hay is being digested. The healthy gut wall of a horse functions as a protective barrier keeping bacteria on the luminal side of the intestine. The ischemic gut wall of a colicky horse, however, is sieve-like, leaky, and no longer impenetrable.

In the poem "Mending Wall," Robert Frost quotes the seventeenth-century proverb "Good fences make good neighbors." Metaphorically, this little piece of wisdom applies to any number of situations in life, including the horse and its gut-flora neighbor.

Havoc ensues as the endotoxin-producing bacteria waste no time in taking advantage of the breach and access the horse's bloodstream. The horse's demise is now imminent.

The bacterial endotoxins trigger the activation of clotting factors and the coagulation cascade. Platelets become activated to form platelet plugs, and blood starts to clot where it's not supposed to. The widespread intravascular coagulation results in the formation of microscopic thrombi that block the networks of capillaries known as capillary beds in critical organs such as the heart, lungs, and kidneys.

The horse's circulatory system is in a free fall as oxygen delivery to critical tissues plummets. The horse's heart beats frantically in an attempt to restore normal blood pressure and quickly approaches a life-threatening level. Cataclysmic multiorgan system failure ensues as a result of the toxic shock.

So how does a veterinarian begin to diagnostically work up the emergency colicky horse?

Let's imagine that you just moved out of the city to the

country. You bought a cute little house on a few acres with a barn, and knowing that it was always your dream to learn to ride, you also bought your very first horse. You bought him from a local horse trader and just couldn't believe how inexpensive he was. You didn't pay too much attention at the time to the fact that his name was Bucky and didn't bother to ask the horse trader how he got the name. You were just thrilled he was such a bargain.

Only a few days after having brought Bucky home, you are on your way down to the barn one evening to do "night check" and you suddenly hear a banging sound coming from the barn. Your pace quickens, since you are obviously anxious to find out what the noise is.

You turn on the barn lights and find that Bucky seems agitated. You notice that he is pawing and realize that the noise you heard was the banging of his hoof against the stall wall as he pawed.

As you open his stall door, Bucky begins to lie down and roll. You see that he didn't finish his hay from the morning feeding, and you quickly sense that something isn't right. You heard about colic in horses somewhere before, and although you aren't quite sure exactly what it is, you suspect that this might be what's going on.

Dashing to the barn phone, you call information to find a nearby equine veterinary practice. Fortunately, there's one fairly close by. You call the clinic and reach the answering service, which is able to patch you through to the on-call veterinarian. You are relieved to hear that they know where your place is and will be there in twenty minutes or so.

The vet pulls up in front of your barn, gets out of his truck, and you thank him for coming out so quickly. He grabs his grip from inside the truck and both of you head inside to find that Bucky is now back up on his feet but beginning to paw once more.

When examining a colicky horse, a horse vet is trying to sort out first and foremost if it's a type of colic that will require surgery.

The exam begins with an assessment of the horse's pain. Is the horse mildly painful or severely so? Is the pain intermittent—in other words does it come and go—or is it relentless and progressive? The level and type of pain that the horse is experiencing is frequently indicative of whether or not the horse will require surgery.

At this point a short-term intravenous pain medication would be given to sedate the horse. The IV meds will cut the pain and relax the horse so that the vet can continue with the exam.

"Hang on to his lead rope," the vet tells you. "I need to slip him a bit of a head hanger," he says as he holds off Bucky's jugular vein and waits for it to distend before giving him an IV injection.

You're wondering what the vet meant when he said something about slipping Bucky a head hanger, when you notice that Bucky already seems much more relaxed. As you watch Bucky begin to lower his head and close his eyes, you realize that the head hanger must have been a sedative.

"Let's have a quick look at his gums," the vet says, pulling Bucky's lip up and pressing his finger against his gums.

You've never seen that done before and are curious as to why the vet wanted to check Bucky's gums. "What can you tell by doing that?" you ask, but realize the vet can't hear you as he already has his stethoscope on and is listening intently to the left side of Bucky's chest.

The color of the mucous membranes and capillary refill

time are a reflection of the horse's blood pressure. Blood pressure has everything to do with vital oxygen being delivered to where it needs to be. In medical jargon, normal blood pressure indicates adequate tissue perfusion.

The color of the gums normally should be pink. Pressing on the gums to see how quickly the color returns after they blanch out is an assessment of the horse's capillary refill time. Try squeezing the tip of your finger until it blanches out, then watch how quickly the pinkish color returns. Color should return within a second or so, and a sluggish return to pink would indicate low blood pressure and likely inadequate oxygenation of tissues.

You're pretty sure that because the vet is listening to the left side of Bucky's chest, he must be listening to his heart, and figure this is the time to sound a bit knowledgeable about what's going on. "How's his heart rate?" you ask. The vet doesn't answer your question but rather says to you, "Hold on just a minute more," and moves the stethoscope from Bucky's chest to seemingly random areas of Bucky's abdomen.

Why would the vet want to listen to Bucky's belly? What's to hear down there? you wonder. You feel a bit confused, as your experience with a physician using a stethoscope has been limited to them listening to your heart and lungs.

"What can you hear in Bucky's belly?" you ask. Without responding, the vet holds a hand up in a "not now" gesture and continues to listen to Bucky's flanks and abdomen.

HMMM . . . PERHAPS I SHOULD INTERRUPT AT THIS POINT. The vet is rather distracted with trying to assess just how colicky Bucky is, and I sense that this is likely why he hasn't answered some of your questions. Let me intervene for a moment and see if I can clear things up.

First of all, the normal heart rate of a horse should be about thirty-six to forty beats per minute. A colicky horse with a heart rate of sixty or more beats per minute is a horse that is likely getting shocky. A heart rate of sixty or more is also a point at which a flag would go up that the horse may need surgery.

"Borborygmi" is the medical term for gut sounds. It's the noise you hear when you're hungry and your stomach rumbles. It's the bubbles and gurgles and sloshing-about sounds of ingesta on the move in a healthy gut. This is what the vet was listening for when he placed his stethoscope over Bucky's abdomen.

Before we go on with the rest of the exam, let's backtrack a bit and chat some more about the degree of pain that the colicky horse is experiencing.

Veterinarians are familiar with the fact that mild come-and-go pain is often associated with a simple obstruction-type colic. Being told that your horse is colicky because it has a simple obstruction is analogous to the ER doc telling you that your abdominal pain is due to the fact that you are constipated. In all likelihood the ER doc would hook you up to an IV, administer some fluids, and have the nurse bring you a glass of water with a tablespoonful or two of a mild over-the-counter laxative such as Metamucil. Lastly, you would probably also get the mini lecture that you need to eat more fiber, drink plenty of liquids, and exercise more.

Horses also become constipated. Veterinarians, however, prefer to use the term "simple obstruction" or "impaction colic" rather than "constipation" when it comes to horses.

Enigmatic is the fact that many horses seem to colic mostly at odd hours of the night. Fortunately, many of these horses with abdominal pain will respond to intravenous pain medication, some oral and/or IV fluids, and a laxative-like compound such as mineral oil.

The horse vet waits and evaluates the horse's response to the medication given. "Does the horse seem more comfortable, relaxed, and pain-free? Can I tell the horse owner that the horse will be fine and that it's okay for them to go back to bed? Or maybe I should tell them to start brewing some coffee."

On the other hand, what if the horse has a twisted piece of gut and needs surgery within the next few hours to survive? Colicky horses that have a piece of strangulating intestine are often those that you can't get to the surgery table soon enough. They often rupture a gut in transit. They never had a chance—peritonitis, septicemia, and toxic shock take them out in the horse trailer.

"WOW, WHAT'S THAT FOR?" you wonder as the horse vet returns from his truck to Bucky's stall with a shoulder-length sleeve.

"Hang on to his lead rope. Here we go," he says as he squeezes some goopy lube onto the sleeve, pulls Bucky's tail to the side, and begins to perform a rectal exam.

The diagnosis of my daughter's acute abdomen was made from an abdominal radiograph taken in the emergency room at our community hospital in the middle of the night. The ER doc pointed out the trapped gas in a portion of her large intestine.

"Why don't you just take an X-ray of the colicky horse's gut to figure out why the horse is colicking?" you ask. Good question, and the answer is really quite simple. X-ray machines powerful enough to see through the belly of the horse hang from ceilings in places like universities and big equine referral hospitals.

Staring somewhat incredulously, you wonder, "What in the world is the vet doing with his arm fully up to his shoulder in Bucky's rear end?"

Bucky is still somewhat sedated as you hold his lead rope. You are correct in assuming that, if not for the sedation, Bucky would certainly not be quite so accommodating about this part of the exam.

At this point, you begin to feel a tad lightheaded and even perhaps a bit shocky yourself at what you are seeing. You're definitely not sure what to think and just have to ask the horse vet, "What exactly are you doing?"

"Oh, sorry, I should have explained," the vet says.

You quickly snap back, "Yes, I wish you would!"

The explanation is not forthcoming, however, as he tells you to "Hang on just a sec longer." With a grimace and then a groan, he pushes his arm in even further. "Hmmm . . . ," you hear him say. "Yup, I think I've got it."

None of this has made any sense to you, and you hear yourself say "Got what?"

"The reason he's colicky, of course," the vet replies.

As the vet takes his arm out of Bucky's rectum and peels off the manure-covered plastic sleeve, he says, "Yup, he's plugged up pretty good. We gotta oil him." Still a bit miffed that no explanation has been given as to what was being done or what the vet actually found or meant by "plugged up," you sense your own blood pressure steadily rising. With frustration but polite restraint you ask, "I'm sorry, but what are you talking about?"

"Be right back," the vet replies, as he heads out the barn to his truck.

It's clear that the vet has incorrectly assumed you were familiar with how a colicky horse is worked up and so didn't bother to go into much detail as to what he did or found. Again, let me provide the explanation that he hasn't.

What can a vet actually feel—or palpate—when he performs a rectal exam on a horse? A lot.

Because the wall of the rectum of the horse has a bit of stretch to it—in other words, because it is pliable—a vet can palpate a lot of what's in the belly of the horse. "Like what?" you ask.

Most of the large intestine is palpable, as are some of the small intestine, the spleen on the left side, the kidneys, bladder, ovaries, uterus, and cervix of the mare. "Wow! That's pretty remarkable," you say. And yes, I would agree.

When stuff goes wrong with what's inside the belly of a colicky horse, this is the single most informative procedure a vet can do. If portions of the intestine are twisted, displaced, distended, or simply obstructed or plugged up, this is most often how equine vets sort out why a horse is colicking.

The veterinarian returns to Bucky's stall carrying a six-foot coiled clear plastic tube. It's called a stomach tube or in medical lingo, a nasogastric tube. The tube is passed up the nostril of the horse to the back of the throat and swallowed by the horse. The tube is then advanced to the stomach, at which point a bilge pump or stomach pump is used to administer medications or a laxative such as mineral oil.

Fortunately, Bucky is still a bit sedated, as most horses are not so keen on what's about to happen.

"Okay, hang on to his halter. Here we go," the vet says to you as he lubes up one end of the stomach tube and inserts it into Bucky's left nostril. Bucky gives a bit of a snort and a toss of his head. The vet steadies his head and reassures him with an “Easy, Bucky, easy now,” and continues to pass the tube to the back of Bucky’s throat. The vet pauses a moment or two and then gives the tube a gentle nudge against the back of Bucky’s throat, causing him to swallow. With one end of the tube in his mouth, the vet blows into the tube every once in a while to dilate the esophagus as he slowly advances the tube down toward Bucky’s stomach.

“If the tube needs to end up in his stomach, why did you put it up his nose?” you ask. Mumbling something unintelligibly, the vet still has one end of the tube in his mouth and casts you another “not now” glance.

I’ll interrupt to answer your question, as the vet seems very much focused on confirming that the stomach tube is in Bucky’s stomach and not his lungs.

Yes, I can see why you would wonder why the vet would put the tube up Bucky’s nose instead of into his mouth if it needs to end up in his stomach. The answer is simple.

First of all, everyone knows that your nostrils eventually lead to the back of your throat where both your windpipe (or trachea) and esophagus are. This is why you can breathe through your nose and also why, when your friend makes you laugh while you’re sipping a soda through a straw, the soda bubbles back out your nose. Putting the tube up Bucky’s nose gets the tube to the same place as putting it in his mouth. The advantage to the nasal route is that Bucky isn’t able to chew on the tube.

“Why did the vet seem so focused when he was passing the stomach tube?” you ask. Good question, and the answer lies in the fact that there is a bit of a potential hazard involved in passing a stomach tube. The vet needs to be sure that the tube is in the esophagus and not in Bucky’s windpipe. The tube needs to end up in Bucky’s stomach and not in his lungs. Imagine pumping three gallons of mineral oil and water into a horse's lungs. Death by drowning would occur within minutes.

The vet reaches for his pail of warm water and mineral oil, attaches the end of the stomach tube to the stomach pump, and pumps the oil and water into Bucky's stomach.

"That should fix him," the vet says as he withdraws the six-foot-long stomach tube out of Bucky's nose. "Turn him out to graze in the morning and wet his hay the next couple of days. Our office will send you a bill."

"I guess he seemed like a pretty good guy," you think to yourself as you watch the vet head out the driveway. Even though you never really got much of an answer to any your questions, you're relieved that Bucky seems comfortable, and it's good to know he'll be okay. You turn off the barn lights and head back up to your house, wondering why Bucky colicked in the first place and how you can prevent him from doing so in the future.

Did you know that drinking plenty of water in and of itself has a laxative-like effect? Veterinarians and ER docs alike wouldn't have to resort to the use of laxatives like mineral oil and milk of magnesia nearly so frequently if horses and people drank more water. This is particularly true for horses, because their diet consists almost entirely of fiber.

Every good horseman knows that the likelihood of colic is much lower in a horse that's a pretty good water drinker, and "Never interrupt a horse while it's drinking" is a frequent admonishment to kids in Pony Club horse management 101.

You remember that the vet instructed you to wet Bucky's hay for a few days and make sure he grazes. Knowing that green grass is mostly water, you conclude that the combination of soaking his hay and grazing him are merely strategies to increase his water intake.

You also realize that what the vet actually meant when he told you that Bucky was plugged up was casual vet lingo for the fact that Bucky was constipated or blocked.

As you reach your house and open the back door to the kitchen, you puzzle about why Bucky colicked so shortly after you brought him home to your barn. Could the move have seemed stressful for him, or has he perhaps just not been drinking enough water? you wonder.

Horses will on occasion forget to drink if they are distracted or stressed, and this often happens shortly after they have moved to a different barn or when they are shipped from home to stable at a show or competition.

Did you know that horses can smell a watering hole half a mile away? This keen sense of smell is of course advantageous for horses in the wild but it makes for a potential problem for horses traveling to a show or track, for example, and here's why: if the water smells at all different at the showground than it does at home, the horse is less apt to drink it.

Knowing that horses can be somewhat finicky about the taste of their water, a good horseman has a few tricks up their sleeve to get a horse to drink more water.

Owners of horses that are shipped frequently will sometimes flavor the horse's water at home with watermelon-flavored Kool-Aid. When the horse is shipped to a show, the Kool-Aid is again added to the water in an effort to disguise any taste differences that the horse might otherwise detect.

Everyone has heard the old adage: You can lead a horse to water but can't make it drink. Yet people have forgotten that the wise old farmer finishes the traditional saying by adding, "but you can salt their oats." And of course, the farmer is right.

Simply adding a couple of tablespoons of salt to the horse's grain every day encourages the horse to drink more water. Imagine sitting down in front of a side order of salty French fries. It wouldn't be too long before you start looking for something to drink.

Bran is another laxative used in horses, and any horse owner worth their salt (pun intended) knows how to mix up a bran mash for their horse. A couple of one-pound coffee cans of bran, a can of sweet feed, and lots of hot water to make a pea-soupy mix is put in the feed bucket. This is a favorite on the menu for horses.

Fifty-pound sacks of bran are found in the feed room of most barns. As you likely well know, oat or wheat bran is a dietary fiber also found in any number of cereal boxes on the supermarket shelves. Bran is a bulk-forming laxative and functions much as a dry sponge does when it becomes wet to hold water.

The laxative-like effects of bran are mild and not nearly as dramatic as the *Saturday Night Live* skit from years ago would have you believe, when they touted a "new" bran-containing breakfast cereal, Colon Blow. Nonetheless, the occasional bran mash given to a horse will help prevent the development of impaction colics by ensuring adequate water intake.

By the way, you have missed out on one of life's simple pleasures if you haven't ever listened to the sound of a horse relishing a bran mash. The nosing around and banging of the feed bucket amidst the slops and slurps will bring a smile into your day.

{SEVENTEEN}

Zonkers Go Bonkers

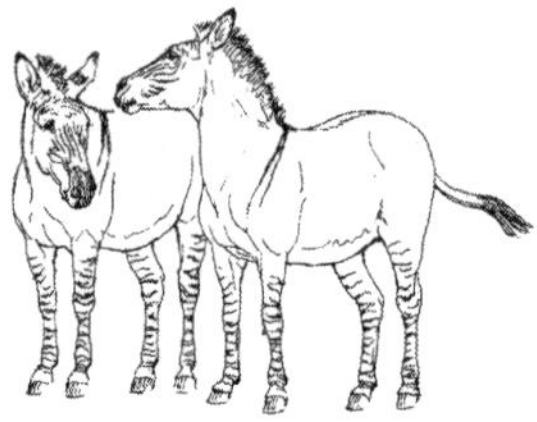

"I THINK YOU BETTER COME AS SOON AS YOU CAN. It's Fred and he got it pretty good from Wilma this time," Jill said anxiously.

"I'm about an hour away just finishing up on a call," I responded.

"Should I give him some bute in the meantime?" Jill asked.

"Good idea, give him a couple of grams and I'll be there as soon as I can," I answered.

The Zonkers had gotten into harmless spats and squabbles in the past during breakfast and dinner but this sounded like more than just horsing around. The last straw actually had more to do with hay, when Wilma became fed up at feeding time and with a quick kick reminded Fred that she was top dog come chow time.

Fred and Wilma Zonkers were actually a couple of "zedonks," the hybrid offspring of a zebra-donkey cross. In crossing zebras with other equids such as a donkey, pony, or horse, a zebra stallion is ordinarily the sire, and the name of the type of offspring describes the equid dam to which the stallion was bred. Zebras bred to horses produce a zorse and the pony cross produces a zonie. Zonked they may seem but with zany zest and zeal zebra zealots seem obsessed in their quest to come up with creative hybrids such as zetlands (offspring of a male zebra and a female Shetland pony), zebrets (male donkey and female zebra), zebrinnys (male horse and female zebra),and zebrules (male zebra and female horse).

All is not equally equid when it comes to the stuff of chromosomes. Donkeys have sixty-two, horses sixty-four, zebras forty-six, and although two genetically different equids can mate, the offspring produced is infertile. An equine equid—a horse bred to a donkey—for example, results in a mule but because the horse has a different number of chromosomes than the donkey, the hybrid offspring is sterile. Similarly, the zedonk hybrid offspring produced when a zebra is mated with a donkey is also sterile.

It's not to say that passion and intimacy were absent from the lives of the Zonkers, but rather that Wilma would forever remain barren and Fred would always be impotent. Nonetheless, the arrival of each new spring and summer would revitalize their hopes, but futile and not fertile would their efforts remain.

The Zonkers were zedonks, the offspring of a zebra-donkey cross and as such displayed traits and characteristics of their parents. Fred and Wilma both had long ears, a hee-haw, and varying strips of striping over parts of their body, but they also had the sometimes unbecoming disposition of both donkey and zebra. Zebras are notoriously quick-tempered and the expression "stubborn as a mule" has a genetic basis in fact, as somewhere encrypted on the donkey chromosome is a rather large strand of DNA having to do with obstinacy.

I headed down the dirt driveway and parked outside the barn. As I hopped out of my truck, grabbing my grip from behind the seat, I heard Jill shout. "We're out here in the paddock behind the barn." "Be right there," I yelled back.

"Hi, Jill, so what happened?" I asked, opening up the paddock gate and noticing that Fred wasn't placing any weight on his right hind leg.

"Well, it started out like most mornings. I threw them each their own pile of hay but of course Fred always thinks her hay is better than his and so he begins to make his way over to hers. Wilma then does her saber-rattling routine, pins her ears, swishes her tail, and fires off a couple of warning shots with a hind leg or two. It's usually right about then that Fred does a one-eighty and goes back to his own pile, but not this time," Jill told me, as I leaned down to examine the swelling in the back of Fred's hind leg.

"It was the craziest thing," Jill added. "The Zonkers have had their little tiffs over breakfast and dinner in the past but this time . . . I don't know. It's as if . . ." Jill paused for a moment, thinking how best to describe the Zonkers' behavior that morning. I didn't want to complete her sentence for her yet I sensed the inevitable.

". . . It's as if they just went bonkers," she said.

"Have him take a couple steps forward," I instructed Jill, wanting to see just how lame Fred was from Wilma's kick to the back of his cannon bone.

Fred reluctantly hobbled forward at a walk, taking several gimpy steps on his right hind leg as Jill tugged on his halter. I knelt down to palpate Fred's cannon bone. "She clocked him pretty good but I don't think there's a fracture," I said.

Easily the most crucial bone in a horse's anatomy is the cannon bone. It's the large bone in each of the four limbs that runs from the knee down to the ankle in the front legs and from the hock down to the ankle in the hind limbs. The long straps of tendon that support and scaffold the front of the cannon bone are called the extensor tendons and those in the rear, which are frequently injured when a horse "bows" a tendon, are the flexor tendons.

"What do you think?" Jill asked.

"Hmmm . . . we're gonna have to do more than just a look 'n feel to see how badly his tendon is injured," I replied, palpating what I suspected to be a partially torn superficial flexor tendon. "We'll have to scan him. C'mon, let's walk him back to the barn and I'll get my ultrasound machine from the truck."

Tendons are stretchy, elastic, and are the tapered ends of muscles anchored to bony insertion sites. When muscles contract, tendinous attachments pull on bone, causing limbs to flex or extend. The microscopic appearance of a tendon is akin to that of the bristles of a paint brush, elastic fibers arranged in parallel so that when a muscle contracts, the fibers pull forcefully as one.

Fred gimped along at a walk as Jill slowly led their way back to the barn. "Here's good, Jill. Let me get set up and we'll have a look," I said, placing my ultrasound machine on a bale of hay and plugging in.

Diagnostic ultrasound machines are used a lot in an equine practice, and being able to scan the ill or injured equine hinges only upon the proximity of an electrical outlet in the barn. That which can be imaged is almost unimaginable, and other than bone and the horse's hoof, just about anything a horse vet wants to see the other side of can be ultrasounded. Preg checks on mares can be done as early as twelve days, the embryonic heartbeat imaged by day twenty-one, and determination of the fetus to be that of a filly or a colt by day fifty-five. The lungs of the horse with pneumonia or pleurisy can be scanned in the barn aisle, and the geriatric pony with the "creaky barn door"–sounding heart murmur can have its faulty heart valves imaged in its box stall. The late-night colicky horse can have its belly scanned stallside to assess the need for colic surgery, and the limbs of the lame can be evaluated while the ultrasound machine rests on a bale of hay.

"What can you see?" Jill asked anxiously, as I knelt down and began scanning the back of Fred's hind leg with the probe of my ultrasound machine.

"Hang on just a sec. Let me have a little better look," I responded and moved the probe back and forth over the area of swelling.

Tendinopathies from overuse are called strains and are associated with overexertion resulting in microscopic tearing of tendon fibers in any number of athletes. Tennis elbow and Achilles tendinitis are common athletic injuries in tennis and basketball players, just as bowed tendons are in racehorses, stadium jumping horses, and dressage horses.

Although overuse tendon injuries may be more frequently seen by physicians and veterinarians, blunt trauma to tendinous structures can be equally if not more crippling. Collisional high-impact tendon-damaging injuries occur in places like football and soccer stadiums and ice hockey rinks—but also in barnyards when ill-tempered zebra types are quick with a kick.

"Jill, it's worse than I thought. There's a blowhole in his superficial flexor that approximates almost the entire diameter of the tendon," I said, staring at the screen of my ultrasound machine.

"What does that mean?" Jill asked uneasily.

"The tendon is almost completely ruptured. Wilma's hoof to the back of his leg near shredded his tendon," I answered, still surprised by what I was seeing on the ultrasound screen.

"Is he going to be okay? What can we do?" she asked.

Veterinary medicine has advanced greatly since *Far Side* cartoonist Gary Larson expressed his view of the perceived limitations of equine therapeutics not that many years ago. His cartoon sketch of an equine veterinary student staring at a list of common horse ailments and the corresponding treatment of each as simply being *"shoot"* insinuated with a bit of both humor and sting an equine vet's restricted options in treating the ill or injured horse at the time.

"If Fred was a racehorse or a jumper, this would have been a career-ender," I said, still scanning his flexor tendon.

"But he and Wilma don't have a career. They don't do dressage, polo, or pull a cart. They're pretty much just lawn ornaments with legs, but I enjoy them so," Jill replied. "I want to do everything we can to help him."

I wiped off the ultrasound gel from the back of Fred's leg and stood up.

"She really blew out his tendon and he may not come fully sound," I told her.

"It doesn't matter, what can we do?" Jill asked.

"It's a touch pricey but it'll get us a better heal than just time and rest," I said. I turned off my ultrasound machine.

"What is it?" Jill asked again.

"We can stem-cell him," I replied.

"Do what?" Jill exclaimed.

If somehow you could microsize yourself and beam down cellside to the debris field of Fred's near ruptured tendon, disarray, chaos, and disaster would stretch out before you. Damage assessment would include the slashed, the mangled, and the crushed, with the once-intact, precisely architected parallel array of microfiber tendinous tissue now appearing hacked, flayed, and tattered. Millions of first responders, the platelets, are already on site by the time you have been transported down and they are frantically at work minimizing further hemorrhage by damaged capillaries.

Overwhelmingly obvious is the fact that a monumental cleanup of carnage will be required before any reparative efforts of the frayed and ragged remnants can begin.

From the vascular system will be deployed militias of giant-size, Pac-Man-like cells called "macrophages," whose job will be to engulf the tissue debris and unidentifiable dead cells, now known simply as "junk-o-cytes." Scar tissue cells—fibrocytes—will eventually arrive and scar in the extraordinary engineering marvel of what once was: the elastic and parallel array of microfibers.

Even the best reparative efforts of fibrocytes, however, to scar in blown-out portions of tendon are far from optimal. The once elastic and resilient stuff of tendinous tissue can only be patched and never truly repaired. Re-injury rates are high in that part of the damaged tendon, because scar tissue doesn't have the capacity to stretch but rather simply tears.

Jill was perplexed. "What do you mean, 'stem-cell him'?"

"Well, it sounds a bit like the stuff of Hollywood but it's

true," I answered.

"What is? What are you talking about?" she asked.

"Stem cells. They're kind of like the robots in that movie *Transformers* that can morph into other objects."

Jill was oddly silent and I sensed I quickly needed to explain further.

"Stem cells have the ability to become almost any type of cell, it just kinda depends on where you put them," I explained.

"But what does that have to do with fixing Fred?" Jill asked.

"Well, if we inject some stem cells into the blowhole in his tendon, they won't exactly turn into new tendon but almost."

"But where would we get them? Don't stem cells come from embryos?" Jill exclaimed.

REGENERATIVE MEDICINE IS AN EMERGING FIELD of sci-fi–like medicine where what once was the stuff of Hollywood is now being researched in medical labs. Doctors specializing in the field of regenerative medicine aren't so much to be found in hospital basements harvesting limbs and organs from humanoids shrouded in cocoons but rather peering into microscopes, strategizing how to use stem cells to regenerate diseased or injured tissues.

"Why patch and repair when you can replace?" is what you might hear a doctor reply when asked about the dizzifying potential of stem cells.

The list of injuries and diseases that the body can't fix, a scalpel can't excise, and medicine can't cure is seemingly endless. The wheelchair-bound with spinal-cord injuries, the stroke victims, those that must undergo daily dialysis because of failing kidneys, the children and the elderly that fill the oncology wards, the blind, the crippled, the autistic, and the depressed are just a few whose lives could be miraculously improved by stem cell therapy.

Stem cells are of two sorts, those that are to be found in embryos and those that are found in adults. Embryonic stem cells are, in medical lingo, highly "undifferentiated" and "pluripotent," which is simply to say that they have super morphing capability and can become any of the 220 different cell types in the adult human body. Harvesting embryonic stem cells, however, destroys the fertilized human embryo, and ethical concerns about this have engendered much controversy in the medical community and elsewhere.

Adult stem cells, however, are found in adults, not embryos, and as such their use skirts any ethical controversy. Adult stem cells are conveniently found in places like bone marrow, but they lack the super morphing potential of embryonic stem cells.

"Hyperdrive" is the name given to certain methods of traveling faster than the speed of light, and "Make it so, Number One" is how Captain Jean-Luc Picard might instruct Commander Will Riker to prepare the Starship *Enterprise* to enter hyperspace to narrowly avoid the villainous Klingons. "Mach one" is the more down-to-earth term used when an Air Force jet such as the F/A-18 Hornet reaches the speed of sound. The speeds of hyperdrive and Mach one are galaxies apart, and therein might lie an appropriate analogy for the comparative morph potential of embryonic stem cells and adult stem cells.

"THEY DON'T ALL COME FROM EMBRYOS. Fred has 'em in his bone marrow," I explained to Jill.

"And how will we get them out and what will they do if we put them in his tendon?" Jill asked.

"TENDINOCYTES" is the name given to the tendon-producing cells that lay down collagen and elastic fibers in a precisely engineered fashion that provides for tendon elasticity and stretch. Adult stem cells, because of their limited morph potential, don't have the ability to mutate into elastic-producing tendinocytes, but they do have the ability to restore a more orderly matrix to the area of injured tendon.

If you were to microscopically examine an area of injured tendon that was allowed to simply scar in, your eyebrows would raise as you adjusted the fine-focus knob on the microscope and zoomed down for a closer look. Jumbled, random, chaotic, and disorganized are adjectives that you might use in describing what you saw. If then you were given a microscope slide of normal tendon tissue to microscopically compare the two, you would likely give a sigh of relief and experience a sense of ease having left the diseased. All would appear orderly, precise, well engineered, and the methodically architected parallel microfibers might suggest a work of art rather than a piece of anatomy.

"LET'S ICE HIM DOWN AND WE'LL GET A GAME PLAN GOING," I said, packing up my ultrasound machine. "Let me check, I think I may have some ice wraps in the fridge in my truck."

"I want to make Fred better as soon as possible. Can we do the stem cell thing right away?" Jill asked.

"HERE WE GO. I did have an ice wrap in the truck," I said to Jill when I returned to the barn aisle. "Here's the game plan. If you can ice down the injury for twenty minutes or so several times a day for the next week, that will help get the swelling down," I added, kneeling down and snugging up the Velcro straps of the ice wrap around Fred's leg. "You'll have to stick him on some bute a couple times a day, which will help with the pain and swelling, but you'll also need to keep him in a stall."

"But what about the stem cell thing?" Jill asked.

"We'll wait a week for the inflammation to quiet down in his tendon and do him then," I said.

It was just about a week later when I pulled down Jill's driveway, parked outside the barn, and began to unload some gear out the back of my vet truck.

I saw Jill coming out of the barn. "How's Fred doing?" I asked her.

"He's still awfully lame. It's heartbreaking to see him in so much pain," she replied.

"Let me get set up and we'll get started," I said. I brought a couple of hay bales over into the barn aisle and laid a few blue surgical towels on top, before placing several vials, needles, and syringes on the makeshift surgery table.

"All right, Jill, I'm just about ready. Bring Fred out into the barn aisle," I said. "Here's the game plan. I'm gonna sedate him some first, block out an area over his chest, and then we'll take the bone marrow aspirate from his sternum," I explained to Jill as I mixed up a triple IV cocktail into a 6 cc syringe.

"Here's the heads-up, however. He's gonna bleed some when I take the bone marrow aspirate," I added as I arranged several instruments, including a scalpel blade, a pair of sterile gloves, a spool of suture material, and the bone marrow trephine on the towels.

"I'm not so sure I'm good with the blood thing," Jill

said, watching me withdraw several milliliters of Carbocaine, a type of local anesthetic, into a syringe.

I slipped a needle into Fred's jugular vein, attached the syringe containing the cocktail, and pushed. "That's gonna *zonk* him pretty good," I said. I withdrew the needle from his vein and glanced at Jill to see if she caught my attempt at a bit of humor.

Within just a few moments of the IV Fred hung his head and began to sway back and forth from the sedation. "That worked pretty fast," Jill noted.

"After we take the bone marrow aspirate, it has to go back to the lab, where they'll isolate the stem cells and then we'll inject them back into his tendon," I explained. I clipped and prepped a small surgical site over Fred's chest with some iodine disinfect.

A trephine is a T-shaped surgical instrument. Its vertical bar is a hollow stainless steel cylinder with saw-like teeth at the base, like a hole saw attachment for an electric drill. The horizontal bar is the handle, which is grasped by the surgeon and, by twisting and applying downward pressure, used to bore out circular sections of bone. There is a crunching sound associated with its use and often the flow of much blood after having bored into the marrow cavity.

"I'm getting a bit faint. I think I need to sit down," Jill remarked as a rather substantial puddle of blood began to form on the barn aisle between Fred's front feet.

"Go ahead, that's fine. I've almost got what I need," I said. I gave another turn, withdrew the trephine, removed the core section of bone marrow contents, and placed it in a sterile vial. "Got it. We're done. I've got a fair bit of marrow," I said. "Let me just suture him up and we can put him back in his stall."

I noticed that Jill seemed a bit pale as she sat on a bale of hay.

Stem cells are good at dividing and reproducing. From the core of bone marrow I removed from Fred's sternum, the lab would isolate the stem cells and, in medical laboratory jargon, expand their population. Fred's bone marrow aspirate likely contained fewer than fifty thousand stem cells, but the lab would isolate those cells, place them on a culture dish, feed them a couple times a day, and within days their population would grow at an exponential rate. I would have millions to inject into Fred's tendon when the lab had done its job.

"All right, Jill, here we go. Hang on to him," I said. It was a week or so later and the lab had called to let me know that Fred's expanded stem cell population was ready. I had stopped by the lab, picked up the vial of ready-to-inject stem cells, transferred them into a syringe, and headed out to Jill's.

"Fred's pretty out of it," Jill commented a minute or so after my having given him a stronger-than-usual IV triple cocktail. I had set up my ultrasound machine on a hay bale, clipped and prepped the area of Fred's tendon injury, taken out an inch-long sterile needle, and knelt down by Fred's right hind leg.

Donkeys don't whinny, horses don't have stripes, zebras lack a hee-haw, and yet they share that which is indeed equally "equid": their ability to kick. They all seem pretty good at it and more often than not, by the time you know it's gonna happen, it's too late.

"He seems awfully wobbly. I think he might fall down. Are you sure you didn't give him too much?" Jill asked.

When it comes to placing needles in the hind legs of equids, equine vets would unanimously agree that less is more. The less sedation given is highly correlated with more of a likelihood of being kicked. I was kneeling down by the hind leg of a bred-to-be-cantankerous zedonk with a good-size needle, about to stick him in a part of his leg that was already hurting.

I held the probe of my ultrasound machine adjacent to the swelling in Fred's hind leg with one hand and with my other, the needle. It was but a flinch and not a kick as I inserted the needle into the skin and deeper.

There on the screen I could see the needle moving as I advanced it closer to the blowhole of Fred's torn tendon. "Thirty million stem cells," the lab tech had said. "And change," he had added with a smile when he handed me the vial.

Like millions of paratroopers parachuting over a war zone, help was on the way, I thought to myself as I attached the syringe of stem cells to the hub of the needle and pushed.

The task would be formidable and time-consuming, lasting perhaps as long as a year. Some would morph into planners, engineers, and architects, but the majority would transform into a vast and unified construction crew.

Tendon injuries are slow to heal because of their poor blood supply and Fred's stem cell therapy wouldn't necessarily buy him a faster heal, just a much better one.

Almost six months would pass before I heard from Jill. "How are the Zonkers doing?" I asked.

"They're both doing so well and Fred is as sound as ever," Jill replied. "It's as if nothing ever happened. In fact after breakfast this morning it was the craziest thing. I don't know what got into them. They were bucking and galloping around the paddock together. It seemed like they just . . ."

Jill paused for a moment, thinking how best to describe the Zonkers' behavior that morning.

{EIGHTEEN}

Roughneck in Lone Star

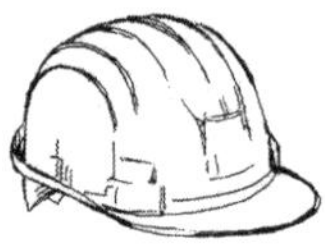

"C'MON KID! MAKE 'EM BITE, MAKE 'EM BITE! I don't give an amadilla's ass if I have to get you out of bed tomorrow with the cat line. We got pipe we gotta get back down there," the driller yelled at me.

The massive diesel engines on the derrick were loud, and I could barely hear him. I clenched my teeth and leaned into the five-hundred-pound pipe wrench tongs to make 'em bite around a new connection of drill pipe. "It's armadillo, not *amadilla*," I wanted to tell him, but he wouldn't have cared anyway.

A string of six thousand feet of drill pipe had to go back into the hole because of a busted drill bit. The chain hand had just thrown a section of chain around the collar of a drill pipe and had taken up the slack using the cathead, an engine-powered rotating drum around which loops of chain or cable are drawn taut.

It was my twentieth birthday. It was also 4:00 a.m. and

I was working the "midnight tower." I was the youngest roughneck in a drilling crew on an oil rig in west Texas, outside the city of El Paso.

The busted drill bit was over a mile down, and more than two hundred sections of thirty-foot drill pipe had to be "tripped out" of the hole, disconnected, and stacked before the roller bit could be changed. The drill floor was slick and noisy, and there were cables and chains that could get ya hurt in a hurry. But the money was good.

The towering structure of an oil rig is designed around a massive block-and-tackle system that can support the weight of more than 250,000 pounds of drill pipe. Down in the hole is the drill bit, which is attached to the end of a string of drill pipe sections, each thirty feet in length. Each section of pipe is threaded at both ends, and the connections have to be made or broken depending on whether the pipe is going in or coming back out.

Tripping out a mile or more of drill pipe to change a drill bit needed everyone working as a team if no one was going to get hurt. I thought we were pretty good at it, even though it seemed I got yelled at more than anyone else. Of the four of us on the drill crew, I was the only one who had all my fingers.

The derrick hand was harnessed in, ninety feet up in the tower, working the end of the drill string as pipe was hoisted out of or lowered into the hole. The drill pipe was stacked upright in slats and, using the "cat line" or cable hoist, it was the job of the derrick hand at the top of the tower to coordinate the lifting or lowering of pipe.

The driller was the head of the crew team and worked the hydraulics, checked gauges, and did a lot of yelling from behind the rotary table on the derrick floor.

The chain hand worked the cat line, a cable hoist, and the cat head. He was also responsible for throwing a loose chain around the collars of drill pipe to make or break pipe connections.

My job as a roughneck was to work with the driller and the chain hand on the drill floor using the tongs, a massive five-hundred-pound pipe wrench of sorts that's suspended by cables, to make or break pipe connections.

A colossal diesel engine the size of a bread truck provided the power to operate the rig. Two other substantially sized diesel engines were also needed, one to provide the electric power on the rig and the other to pump "mud" down the hole.

If I wasn't on the drill floor making or breaking pipe connections, my job as a roughneck included mixing a lot of cement-size bags of mud. Mud on a drilling rig isn't the same stuff you scrape off the bottom of your boots, it's a chemical slurry that's mixed, stored in tanks, and pumped down the hole to lubricate the drill pipe and bit.

The noise of the engines on the drill floor was near deafening. We had to shout to be heard, and I would attribute my partial loss of hearing in what I would later call my "trick left ear" to the six months I worked on the oil rig.

"Ya comin', kid?" the driller asked me.

"Be right there," I answered. I got out of my coveralls and hung my hard hat up. It was 7:30 A.M.; our shift was over and another crew had already arrived. We all piled into the driller's dust-covered Bonneville for the hour-long drive back to El Paso.

"Good job, kid," the chain hand said from the front seat, handing me an icy-cold can of Lone Star beer.

I was hot, dirty, and we were doing ninety miles an hour

with the windows open along Interstate 10. I sipped on the icy beer and agreed with the nodding donkeys or pumpjacks I saw out the window—the breeze felt good.

El Paso is like a lot of other parts of Texas, one of those places that looks better in the rearview mirror, but I needed the money. My room at Motel 6 was six dollars a night back then, and huevos rancheros was what I usually ate at Rosa's Cantina, a Tex-Mex truck stop in town. And the armadillo is still the state animal of Texas.

I had left Bombay to go to Istanbul and then on to North Africa, where I was promptly detained when I arrived in Casablanca. I was led into the immigration office by a couple of Moroccan soldiers with machine guns who instructed me to sit on a chair in a small room with a desk and a framed picture of King Hassan wearing a red fez with blue tassels.

The machine gun–toting soldiers returned with an immigration official whose English was as good as my Arabic. "*Parlez-vous français?*" he asked me. Fortunately, French is Morocco's second language, and I had taken seven years of it in elementary and boarding school. "*Oui, un peu. Quel est le problème?*" I responded. "*Nous ne pouvons pas vous permettre d'entrer dans notre pays* à *moins que vous vous coupiez les cheveux. Tenez, c'est une paire de ciseaux.*"

I had been handed a pair of scissors and told that I would not be allowed to enter the country unless I cut my hair. I guess I could see his point. I must have appeared somewhat scraggly. The cook in Australia had last cut my hair and it had been at least six months since.

I sat in the chair in front of him and cut my hair until he nodded, after which he stamped my passport. I left the airport and took a bus into the part of Casablanca known as the Old Medina near the harbor in the open-air souk, or market, and found a street barber to finish what I had started. I bought a djellaba—striped it was—and a pair of sandals and spent the next few months practicing my French, enjoying couscous, and escaping the desert heat by trekking in the Atlas mountains.

I was still searching for my dad in many ways. The last time I had seen him was when I was eight years old. My quest, however, was not about finding him in the literal sense of discovering where he had moved to, but more about understanding the journey to be a man. Growing up those many years without a dad left a void and a vacuum of sorts in my life as to what a man is supposed to be and do. I finished boarding school at age seventeen and the following three-year journey of self-discovery wasn't a planned itinerary designed to take me around the world and land me in El Paso, but it did.

In Morocco I would later meet my runaway sister in Tangiers, and together we would spend some time traveling in Europe before I left to visit a classmate from boarding school in South America. His family owned a *hacienda ganadera* or cattle ranch near Lake Maracaibo in western Venezuela. They were also big in brewing and owned Cerveza Polar, the largest brewery in Venezuela.

My time spent in Venezuela visiting my friend's cattle ranch included a few days with a *veterinario equino*—or horse vet—where I saw the bulldozing of twenty or so swamp fever–positive horses in a trench burial.

America is very different from the rest of the world. We are protected from much. The diseases of cattle and horses that veterinarians in America mostly only read about are a daily reality in Latin America and elsewhere.

Equine infectious anemia (EIA, or swamp fever) is a viral disease of horses transmitted by mosquitoes. It is stringently tested for in the USA, where in fact horses are required to have a negative Coggins test for EIA antibodies in the blood in order to compete or travel in America and abroad. There is no cure for EIA. An infected horse remains so for life and becomes a potential reservoir of infection for other horses. Quarantine is impractical. In twenty-five years as a veterinarian in the United States, I have never seen a horse test positive. And yet, in a single day in Venezuela I saw twenty horses buried.

My Venezuelan classmate from boarding school was one of the elite, the super-rich, and his older brother had his own plane. From Caracas, the Venezuelan capital city, we flew to the Dutch-owned island of Curaçao just off the coast. The landing strip was a local beach, and we spent the afternoon eating mangoes, melons, and fresh fish.

Rickety bus trips, however, were how I made my way through Panama, Costa Rica, Nicaragua, Honduras, Guatemala, and Mexico to Chihuahua and the city of Juarez.

"The pass" from the border city of Juarez, Mexico, into the United States is the city of El Paso, Texas. I walked into a drilling company the next day and was hired as a roughneck, which is how I would spend the next six months of my life.

Perks and benefits weren't discussed, OSHA wasn't around, workers' comp didn't exist, and health insurance was never mentioned. It was just about the money. In the oil fields of west Texas, if you got hurt, you lost your job. It was a seven-day-a-week job, and if a roughneck wanted time off, he had to quit, rest up, and go get rehired.

The sun had come up an hour or so ago and I was mixing

mud. A geologist from the drilling company had come out that morning to run some tests on core samples taken at the rig, and I became curious as to what he was doing.

"My dad is a geologist too," I told him. I talked and he listened. It was really the first time anyone had asked me about my life and what I thought I was going to do with rest of it.

"So what are you thinking that you want to do?" the geologist asked me.

"I'm not sure. What did your dad do?"

"He was a cow vet outside Wichita Falls," the geologist told me. "He was real good at it, he enjoyed working with the ranchers, and I went on calls with him lots."

"So why didn't you want to become a vet?" I asked him.

"I almost did. I liked working with the cattle, the ranchers, but just not the hours," he said. "I enjoy being a geologist. It's interesting, I travel some, and about the only emergency call I might get is if we had an earthquake," he added jokingly.

We talked some more about our dads, my travels, about doing something in life that makes a difference for good, and the opportunities in life that an education provides.

I quit my job on the oil rig the next day, wanting to go to college.

{NINETEEN}

Chocolate Kisses

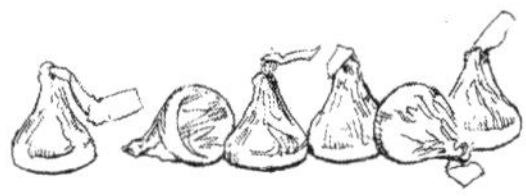

IT WAS A BEAUTIFUL BLUE-SKY DAY IN JUNE. I had just finished suturing up a horse that needed several stitches after snagging his nostril on a gate latch, and I was thinking about a cup of coffee when my cell phone went off.

"Doc, you gotta come right quick. One of my best show horses is down and I can't get him up." Ordinarily Courtney was fairly calm when a horse was injured or colicky but this time she sounded panicky. "I'm twenty minutes away, Courtney, tell me what's going on."

"It's my daughter's paint show horse Hershey. We were getting ready to take him back for a second day at a horse show this afternoon and while we were grooming him on the barn aisle he suddenly went down. We can't get him up."

I turned down the driveway of Hay in the Hair Farm and saw Courtney standing outside the barn waiting for me. "Hi, Courtney, what happened?" I asked as I climbed out of my truck and opened up the side cabinets.

"He's still down on the barn aisle. He was on the cross ties while my daughter was grooming him when he just collapsed. We've been trying to get him up but he won't move."

I grabbed my stethoscope and a thermometer and headed toward the barn with Courtney. "What do you mean he just collapsed? Did he seem colicky before he went down?" I asked.

"No, not at all. He's been fine," Courtney said. "When I went to catch him up out of his paddock he walked over to the gate as he usually does, and we haltered him up, brought him into the barn, and put him on the cross ties. All of a sudden he kinda sat down like a dog on his haunches, busted the cross ties, and laid down right there on the aisle. I've never seen anything like it."

"Let's take a look," I said.

We turned down the barn aisle to find Hershey lying motionless on his side on the floor of the aisle. "You remember Hershey—he was the foal that was born a little early and wasn't strong enough to nurse on his own for a couple of days. You had to come out and leave a stomach tube in him taped to his halter so we could feed him every couple of hours," Courtney said.

"It's been a couple of years but I remember. How old is he now?" I asked.

"He just turned three this June," Courtney responded.

Hershey lay quietly on the concrete aisle floor staring up at me as I knelt down by his side and stroked his neck. I stood up, gave a couple of clucks and a tug on his lead rope, but Hershey made no attempt to move. "We‘ve been trying that, Doc, he won't even try. It's like he's paralyzed,"

Courtney said.

"Tell me what happened again, Courtney," I said.

"It was the weirdest thing. We were just grooming him up on the cross ties and Hershey just kinda sits down on his haunches and then sort of falls over on his side."

"Did he slip?" I asked.

"No, he didn't slip. It happened all of a sudden."

Clearly something was very wrong. Anyone who has spent any time around horses knows that it's just not in a horse's nature to lean back, break a set of cross ties, and suddenly lie down in a barn aisle. It's not to say that horses won't lie down on occasion, but usually it's in the confines of a bedded stall or perhaps out in the paddock and, I might also add, only when they feel it is safe to do so.

I walked behind Hershey and knelt down. "Let me check his temp," I said to Courtney. When I lifted his tail and inserted the thermometer, the anal reflex was absent. This was odd. The normal reaction to a thermometer being placed in the anus of a horse is that the anal sphincter reflexively pooches out. It's a reflex, a bit like the knee-jerk reaction, or patellar reflex, when a physician taps your knee with a tendon hammer.

"His temp is normal, no fever," I told Courtney. "But it's odd that his tail is flaccid and his anal reflex is missing when I put the thermometer in."

"What's that mean?" Courtney asked.

"I'm not sure quite yet," I said.

I knew that a flaccid tail and a lax anal sphincter tone was something seen with spinal-cord trauma, but there was no history or indication of a fall or injury. Besides, even if Hershey had somehow slipped and fallen when he was turned out and injured his spinal cord, he certainly wouldn't have been able to walk from the paddock into the barn when Courtney brought him in.

I also knew that an infection of his spinal cord by a bacteria or virus resulting in an encephalitis or meningitis might also result in a flaccid tail, but Hershey would have been running a fever, and typically there would have been more of a gradual onset of clinical signs.

"What do you think is wrong?" Courtney asked.

I didn't answer as I really didn't know. "Let me have a listen," I said, as I knelt back down and placed my stethoscope over Hershey's chest. His heart rate was slightly elevated as was his respiratory rate but both insignificantly so. I pretended to continue to listen as if I was onto something but really I was scrambling for more time to sort out what was going on, when Courtney interrupted. "You see that, Doc? It looks like he's starting to twitch some."

Courtney was right. We both watched as what started out as an occasional muscle twitch in Hershey's shoulder quickly began to progress and affect more of his muscles along his neck and back. "Why is he starting to twitch like that? What's wrong with him?" Courtney asked.

"I don't know, Courtney, but let's make him a bit more comfortable. Can you bring a saddle pad to put under his head?" I asked.

In the minute it took for Courtney to return with a saddle pad, Hershey's entire body was in tremors. "Doc, he's getting worse. Why is he shaking like that? Is he having a seizure? What's he doing?" she exclaimed in an almost panic.

"I'm not sure. I just don't know yet but let's get this saddle pad under his head," I said.

When I picked up Hershey's head to position the saddle

pad, it was as if he was unconscious but wide awake at the same time. His body from head to tail seemed limp but his eyes were wide open, staring helplessly, almost pleadingly at me.

My mind was racing, trying to sort out what was wrong with Hershey. I had never seen anything like this before. It all seemed to happen so quickly. He was apparently fine one minute and then in a state of dishrag paralysis and tremors the next.

Muscle fasciculations, or tremors, are frequently the result of electrolyte imbalances. However, the horse is usually stiff, reluctant to move, still standing and not down. "Tying up" is the appropriate name given to one of these electrolyte disorders that result in the horse becoming rigid and unwilling to move, almost as if they are in fact tied up. Hershey, on the other hand, seemed limp, weak, and not so much unwilling to move as unable to move.

"Has anything changed in the last few days like his diet, his routine, his turnout, anything you can think of that might be different?" I asked.

"Everything has been the same other than we took him to a horse show yesterday and were planning to go again today," Courtney answered.

"Are your other horses okay?" I asked.

"They're all fine," she told me.

"What did Hershey do at the horse show?" I asked.

"It was a halter show and we were only there for a couple of classes," Courtney said. "He loaded right up on the trailer and seemed fine once we were there."

"How old is Hershey now?" I asked her.

"I told you earlier: He just turned three this June," she responded.

"Sorry, I'm just trying to go over everything in my mind." I thought for a minute. "What do you feed him?" I asked.

"He's on an alfalfa-molasses mix with a couple pounds of sweet feed," she replied.

"And you have other horses on the same ration?" I asked, trying to determine if somehow the paralysis was a feed-related toxicity.

"The other horses are all pretty much receiving the same feed and they're all fine," Courtney answered.

I knew that botulism can cause the shakes and paralysis in horses, but because the toxin is often associated with contaminated grain or hay, more than one horse is usually affected.

"Hang on a sec, I'll be right back," I said, trying to sound purposeful and knowing. I stood up and headed back to my truck. I was drawing a blank as to what could be wrong. I needed a few minutes, but more than time I needed a silver bullet, a magic potion or vial of "injectafix" to come sprinting back with from my truck.

"What could cause such a rapid onset of paralysis and tremors?" I thought to myself. I ran down a list of possible causes in my mind, but everything I could think of either had more of a gradual onset or somehow just didn't seem to fit. Toxins in the feed would likely have affected the other horses and there was no history or indication of trauma that might have resulted in a vertebral fracture. Rabies would have come on more gradually and an encephalitis or meningitis would have had an accompanying fever spike.

I slid open the drawer in the back of my truck and stared at the fifty or sixty vials of injectable medications. "C'mon think, think, figure it out. What's wrong with him?"

Hershey's sudden paralysis and tremors didn't seem like any kind of neurological disorder I had seen in the past nor any type of poisoning or toxicity I had encountered before.

"Doc, hurry up, he's shaking pretty bad," Courtney yelled from inside the barn.

"I'm coming," I yelled back. I grabbed a pair of clippers, some betadine disinfect, alcohol, a catheter, a vial of Valium and some syringes, needles, and blood tubes.

I knelt down and slipped a 19-gauge needle into Hershey's jugular vein, attached the syringe of 40 mg of Valium, and pushed. "That will stop the shaking," I explained.

"Have you ever seen this happen before?" Courtney asked as we watched and waited for the Valium to take effect.

"I haven't, but let me take some blood for a CBC and chem panel," I said, and began swabbing down Hershey's jugular vein with an alcohol swab.

"What are we going to do? Do you think he'll be okay?" Courtney asked.

"Here's the game plan," I said. "All I can figure is that Hershey must have some sort of electrolyte disorder. We'll get a catheter in and give him a bunch of IV fluids and hope that fixes him."

Limp was Hershey and limp-sounding was what the owner must have thought of my game plan. "Give him a bunch of fluids and hope that fixes him" sounded more like a salvage plan, last-ditch and likely as reassuring as if I had just told her to start buying his hay one bale at a time.

I took some blood samples but there was no white-coated lab tech to hand them off to who could have disappeared down a hall to run a stat chem screen and CBC. I would have to take the blood samples back to the clinic and turn them in to a diagnostic lab and wouldn't have results until the next day.

Could something have happened at the horse show? I wondered. This was unlikely, I concluded, as Hershey was a halter horse and would have competed in a class where the horses are led and shown in hand and not ridden. Halter horses aren't performance horses. They get lined up and looked at. They don't break a sweat galloping, jumping, or chasing down steers at a rodeo. The likelihood of an injury or exertion-induced electrolyte imbalance sustained while standing in a line with other horses in a conformation class would be slim to none.

The Valium kicked in. Hershey's shakes had quieted down by the time I got out my clippers and began to shave up an area over his jugular vein. No sooner, however, had I started to scrub up the clipped area with some betadine and alcohol when Courtney asked, "What's he doing with his eyes?"

I looked at Hershey's eyes and saw that the nictitating membrane, or third eyelid, was partially drawn across both eyes.

"That's odd. That's his third eyelid coming across his eyes."

"Why's he doing that, Doc?" she asked.

"I don't know. It could be the Valium I gave him but I've never seen that happen before," I answered.

"Is Hershey gonna be okay?"

"I wish I could tell you that I knew he was, but I just don't know," I admitted.

Sometimes wrong but never in doubt was the strategy preached when I was in veterinary school. Act and talk like you know what you're doing even if you sometimes don't was the drift. Brimming with bravado, however, was not how I was feeling: So far the only answers I had managed to come up with were a lot of "I don't knows." I was at a loss and bewildered by what could be wrong with Hershey, and Courtney was likely feeling as reassured about Hershey's outcome as I was confident about knowing how to treat him.

"We're in," I said, as a flash of blood appeared in the hub of the catheter. I slid the rest of the catheter into Hershey's jugular vein, withdrew the six-inch needle stylet, and capped off the end of the catheter.

"I'll be right back. Let me get some fluids and an IV line from my truck," I told Courtney and headed out the barn. Behind the seat of my truck I kept thirty to forty liters of Ringer's solution. I grabbed a couple of the five-liter bags and an IV line and returned to the barn.

"We'll run some fluids to him and hope that fixes him, but we're gonna have to figure a way to sling him if he doesn't get up soon," I told Courtney.

"What do you mean?"

Horses sleep standing up for good reason. A complicating problem which I had yet to mention to Courtney would soon arise from the fact that a horse that is down for more than an hour or so is a horse that is less and less likely ever to be able to stand back up on its own.

"Compartment syndrome" is a severe muscle-related disorder that results from compression to the down muscles of twelve hundred pounds of horse that can't get up. Because the connective tissue that surrounds muscle bundles doesn't stretch, swelling of the muscles that are being compressed by the weight of the horse above causes pressure to rise greatly in the muscle space, or "compartment." A life-threatening condition develops within just hours of a horse being down as inflammation, lack of blood flow, nerve damage, and edema soon develop in the muscles being compressed.

I had to sling many horses in the past that couldn't get back to their feet for whatever reason, using belly bands and the likes of hoists, pulleys, and the front end loader of tractors.

Fortunately, horses have the ability to lock their joints, which anatomically enables them to sleep standing up. Of course, this is hugely advantageous for their survival in the wild, allowing them to flee from the attack of would-be predators at a moment's notice. The few seconds it would take for a horse in the wild to rise to its feet from the much too vulnerable position of lying down might be the fateful advantage a mountain lion or pack of coyotes in search of a meal would need.

"All right, Courtney, here we go," I said as I hooked the IV line up to the catheter in Hershey's neck and started to run the fluids. "It'll take about forty-five minutes to run the ten liters of Ringer's."

Muscle cramping and tremors are often associated with dehydration and electrolyte depletion as a result of prolonged exertion and sweating. Marathon runners hold out a hand and grab a banana on the run every several miles to replenish lost potassium. Unfortunately, racetrack and cross-country horses are not so, hmmm . . . shall we say, handy?

Fluid therapy accounts for several chapters in any medical pharmacology textbook, and for good reason. It is often the single most lifesaving procedure in horse and human patients alike suffering from fluid or blood loss caused by dehydration, trauma, shock, surgery, or severe burns.

An English physician by the name of Dr. Ringer placed very precise quantities of sodium chloride (common salt), potassium chloride, and calcium chloride in water and developed a sterile, balanced, and isotonic solution.

"Sterile," of course means that the fluids are free of any microorganisms. "Balanced" means that the acid–base balance—or pH—of the fluid is identical to that of blood, neither acidic nor alkaline but neutral. And "isotonic" means that the fluids to be administered intravenously also contain the same salt concentration as blood cells.

Hooking someone up to an IV and running just water into their bloodstream would result in the person's death in about five or six minutes. "Massive hemolysis" would be included somewhere on the coroner's report.

A simple law of chemistry is that water follows sodium. Because all cells, including blood cells, contain sodium chloride in their normal chemical composition, water would move by diffusion into the red blood cells, causing them to rupture, or hemolyze.

Courtney and I silently knelt by Hershey's side as the last liter of the first bag of fluids began flowing. Hershey still remained motionless and limp. I was discouraged and of course knew that Courtney was even more so. We both sensed that surely there should have at least been some improvement if we were on the right track in treating him for an electrolyte imbalance.

"Let's get him started on the other bag," I said. I switched the IV line over to the second five-liter bag, hung it up on the cross tie screw, knelt back down by Hershey's side, and stroked his neck.

In a somewhat similar way to how chemical reactions in your car battery result in the generation of electricity to start your car, muscle cells use the positive charges of sodium, potassium, and calcium to set up electrical potentials that allow muscle cells to contract.

How muscle cells actually contract so you can lace up your riding boots, put a foot in the stirrup, and swing a leg over the saddle involves a bit of biochemical wizardry. Taking up the reins requires a delicately designed constellation of biochemical reactions that not only converts sugar and fat to muscle fuel but also generates electricity as voltage-gated sodium channels in muscle cells open and close.

"What am I missing? What don't I see?" I thought to myself as I stared at Hershey. The second five-liter bag was half-empty and he was still lying as limp as a dishrag.

"Tell me more about Hershey," I said to Courtney. "Is he a good guy?"

A smile came over Courtney's face. "Well of course, that's how he got his name. He's been such a sweetie ever since he was a foal. He was easy to name, just as kind and sweet as they come. His sire is a fancy muscled-up halter horse that did real well on the show circuit."

"What's the stallion's name?" I asked.

"He's a stud out in Oklahoma. Impressive is his name, and if you saw his show record he is just that—pretty impressive."

I glanced up at the almost-empty second five-liter bag of Ringer's solution and followed the IV line down to where it attached to the catheter. I was staring at the catheter lost in thought, trying to recall something I had read in one of my veterinary journals about a stallion that had some genetic disorder affecting his offspring.

"It's what Courtney said about Hershey's muscled-up sire," I thought to myself. "It was the name of the stallion . . . Of course, that was it . . . how to treat Hershey had everything to do with his name!"

Courtney nudged me. "Hey, Doc, the bag is empty."

"Sorry, I wasn't listening. What'd you say?" I asked.

"The bag's empty. Now what?"

I jumped up excitedly and smiled. "Courtney, you're right. Hershey is a sweetie and guess what? He's about to become even more so!" I exclaimed, heading out of the barn.

"Where are you going?" Courtney yelled.

"Don't move, I'll be right back," I said.

"Don't worry, Hershey isn't going anywhere," Courtney shouted back somewhat sarcastically.

I raced out to the truck and slid open the back cabinet again. Scanning the vials of medication frantically, I thought to myself, "Where is it? I know I've got some."

It flashed through my mind that the ten liters of fluids I had just given Hershey was actually making matters worse, but that didn't matter now. Hiding way back of meds I hadn't used for a while was a 500 cc bottle of IV dextrose. "Got it! I did have the injectafix after all," I thought.

"Doc, what's that?" Courtney asked as I hooked up the bottle of dextrose to the IV line and watched the syrupy mix flow down toward the catheter in Hershey's jugular. "I'm hoping a couple of glug-glugs of this stuff will do it," I said excitedly.

"Lock 'n load, Hershey—here it comes," I said, and I opened the catheter port wide open. "He's getting sweeter by the moment now," I told Courtney. "This stuff is basically an IV sugar solution, and if we're a little lucky, he'll be okay."

"How is sugar gonna fix him?" Courtney asked.

"Give me the lead rope and let's stand back some," I said as I saw the last of the dextrose solution run down the IV line.

Hershey lay there and watched us step back. It was time. I gave a couple of clucks and a tug on the lead rope, and Hershey just sort of rolled up on his sternum, gave a snort like he was blowing off a bad dream, and jumped to his feet.

"He's okay! I can't believe he's all right!" Courtney said, putting her arms around Hershey's neck.

Hershey was the first and most memorable case of "Impressive syndrome" that I would encounter.

The syndrome is actually a genetic disorder affecting the descendants of the Quarter horse sire Impressive. Over the years, the stallion's buff and beefy offspring cleaned up in the halter horse show ring world, which of course led to his extensive use at stud. Tragically, by the time the mysterious genetic mutant DNA that controls the sodium channels in muscle cells was identified as originating from the stallion, thousands and thousands of Quarter horses, Appaloosas, and paint horses would be affected.

Hyperkalemic periodic paralysis, or HyPP, is the more correct medical term for Impressive syndrome. It results in dangerously high levels of blood potassium, thought to be brought on by transportation or stress.

Hershey actually did have an electrolyte disorder, one that I was inadvertently making worse by giving him the Ringer's solution, which contained additional potassium.

Encrypted on the defective DNA of Impressive's offspring is a faulty cellular switch regulating the flow of sodium and potassium in and out of the muscle cells. The outpouring of potassium into the blood, medically termed hyperkalemia, interferes with the muscle cells' ability to contract. Sodium channels open excessively and the muscle is prone to be more easily excited, which is often observed as muscle fasciculations. As the cellular floodgates open and potassium spills out into the circulation, the ability of the muscle cells to contract is lost altogether, causing the horse to develop a flaccid paralysis.

Oddly enough, treatment consists of raising the horse's blood glucose, which lowers blood potassium levels by driving the potassium back into the muscle cells. A couple of ounces of Karo syrup squirted into the mouth is the cheap and effective fix for a horse in the incipient stages of an attack. A horse like Hershey, however, that was down and limp needed the IV dextrose.

I called Courtney later in the day to check in on Hershey and go over a game plan of sorts as to how we could best manage a disorder he would have for the rest of his life. She would have to avoid feeds that were high in potassium, like alfalfa and molasses, and Hershey would have to take a couple of water pills, or diuretics, every day to help him eliminate potassium in his urine. Courtney would also now have to add to her emergency kit in the barn a bottle of Karo syrup.

I was heading home from a call in San Simeon, driving south along the Pacific Coast Highway. The foothills and canyons along the central coast of California in June are wonderfully golden, the arroyos and gulches dry, and the cattle in the heat of the day to be found milling about in the shade provided by the groves of minty-smelling eucalyptus trees.

I turned up my clinic driveway and parked outside the exam barn to find a package with a note by the door. The note simply read: "Thanks Doc." Inside the package was a bag of bite-size chocolates, teardrop-shaped and flat-bottomed, all individually wrapped in silver foil. You know the ones—Hershey's Kisses.

{TWENTY}

Rhinos and Tigers and Gorillas, Oh My!

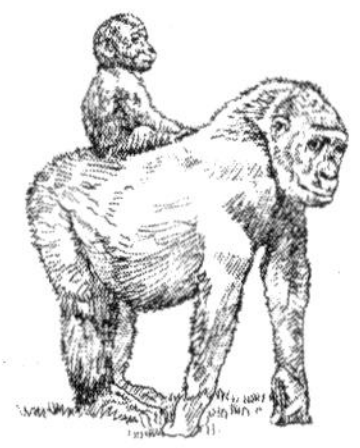

"HEY, DOC, IT'S LULU, she just broke her water and is going into labor," Tom said.

It was late on a Friday evening and I was almost asleep when my cell phone went off. "I'm on my way. Can you call the others and let them know?" I said, hopping out of bed.

I didn't need to sift through any questions. Tom was good and knew when to call.

Lulu was on the critically endangered list, due any day, and we had anticipated there might be a problem. The last ultrasound we performed only a few days ago revealed a placenta previa: the afterbirth was in front of the cervix, a complication that was life-threatening to mom and baby. Lulu would require a Caesarean section.

It had been a group decision to wait. Rather than induce labor with an injection of Pitocin (the hormone oxytocin) as is frequently done in humans, we decided to wait for Lulu to go into labor on her own and then perform the Caesarean section.

It was my first year out of veterinary school and I was an intern in the large-animal clinic at Ohio State University's veterinary school. Most of my classmates had decided to go right out into practice but I had chosen a different direction, that of an internship and a residency.

I knew I wanted to work just with horses, so a large-animal internship was a step in the right direction. I wouldn't be sidetracked by having to work with cats, dogs, or birds and the additional three years of training would allow me the opportunity to focus on my interest in equine medicine.

OSU's veterinary school was one of the first in the United States. The state is big into farming and livestock, and when I applied for the year-long large-animal internship position, I was under the assumption that "large animal" was limited to the likes of horses, beef and dairy cattle, hogs, and perhaps the occasional llama.

My dream of wanting to work exclusively with horses, however, would have to wait. The description of the large-animal internship on the application somehow omitted mention of the array of other "large animals," including Lulu, a three-hundred-pound western lowland gorilla at the Columbus Zoo.

My life for the next year would be altogether different from what I had anticipated, very much serendipitous, and at times filled with surprise. I would indeed have the opportunity to work with horses but also with an unexpected assortment of large animals, from lame elephants and zebras to pregnant giraffes, rhinoceroses with diarrhea, and a cranky tiger with a toothache.

Tom was a zookeeper and happened to walk in on Lulu and her male companion Congo during an evening of intimacy and embrace eight and half months ago, the gestation length of western lowland gorillas.

It was now close on midnight and Tom was waiting for me as I pulled up outside the primate center and jumped out of my truck. "Hey, Tom, how's Lulu doing?" I asked, grabbing my grip from behind the seat.

"I called just as soon as I saw her break her water," Tom replied.

"And what about Congo, did you have a chance to move him into the adjacent cage?"

"Yeah, I did, but it wasn't easy. He just about went ape when I separated him from Lulu," Tom replied with a smile. "The others are on the way but they told me we should get started as soon as you arrived," Tom added.

"We'll leave the lights off so as not to disturb the rest," Tom said as we opened the door to the gorilla house. We each stepped into the footbath of disinfect before going any further. It was dark but I could hear them. The rest of the troop was supposed to be asleep but they were restless and somehow sensed the time had come.

The smell of gorilla is thick and sweet. I could feel them watching us as we walked along the dimly lit hallway and down some steps that led into the prep room. It was a large room with tables, counters, and bins of fruit and vegetables. This was where meals were made and also where an assortment of medications such as antibiotics and anti-inflammatories for some of the gorillas were mixed and added to bottles of fruit juice.

Gorillas are susceptible to a lot of the same ailments that humans encounter, including respiratory infections like the flu, intestinal disorders such as bacterial enterocolitis, and any number of arthritic conditions. I had to have a TB test as an intern before I could work at the zoo and was reminded not to work with any of the primates if I had a cold or the flu.

"They'll be here soon," I said, looking at my watch. "We should get started." I opened up my grip and took out a bottle of Ativan.

Tom reached for a ripe mango from one of the bins. "This is her favorite," he said. I handed Tom a couple of 10 mg tabs of Ativan, a Valium-like drug that Lulu would receive as a pre-anesthetic. Tom tucked the Ativan tabs into a slice of mango and headed over to Lulu's cage door.

Zoos have changed a lot over the years; their exhibits have become more natural, elaborate and akin to the wildlife's actual habitat. Lulu's cage door opened up into what was really more of a bedroom, a relatively private area from which she could wander out into a lush green jungle-like expanse that she shared with the rest of the troop. It was only in the last few weeks of her pregnancy that she had been partitioned off from the others so that Tom could keep an eye on her.

Gorillas are social animals and as such Lulu and her mate Congo shared a bedroom until the last month or so of Lulu's pregnancy. Lulu had recently made it clear to Tom that she felt agitated when Congo bothered her at night and she would prefer that they sleep in separate bedrooms. Tom acceded to Lulu's request despite the evening ritual objections and antics of Congo at the change in sleeping arrangements.

Lulu was a big girl and enjoyed her diet of about thirty pounds of fruit and vegetables a day. She was fifteen years old now and had been rescued from the ravages of a war-torn Republic of Angola in southern Africa, where her mother died when Lulu was only two years old.

The twenty-five-year-long Angolan Civil War spawned a devastating crisis on millions of people and also upon the mountain and lowland gorillas of Angola, Zambia, and Republic of the Congo. Fortunately, Lulu wouldn't become a casualty of war as had her mother but rather would enjoy a life of peace and safety, likely living to be fifty years old or more in the Columbus Zoo.

Lulu's coat was short, soft, fine, and very much unlike those of the mountain gorillas that live at higher elevations, whose coats are thick and shaggy. She stood five feet tall and weighed close on three hundred pounds, having put on a few extra pounds living in the comfort and safety of the zoo.

"Here you go, girl," Tom said to Lulu, opening her cage door and handing her the Ativan-laced slice of mango.

"That'll start to take effect in about fifteen minutes," I said. "They'll be here soon. Let's get the other stuff ready."

The thought of a gorilla on a gurney being wheeled through the hallways of "labor and delivery" at the university hospital seemed to alarm some of the hospital administration officials. An alternate plan brought smiles and relief, however. We would borrow some equipment from the departments of OB/GYN and pediatrics to bring to the zoo, where we improvised a surgery suite in the corner of the prep room.

Tom and I wheeled out a gurney, placed the bassinet and incubator off to the side, and set up the ventilator and several tanks of gas that would be used as part of the inhalant anesthesia. There was a tank of isoflurane, a tank of nitrous oxide (laughing gas) and a couple of tanks of oxygen. The triple blend of gases would be used to maintain Lulu in a state of general anesthesia throughout the operation. Another general anesthetic, however, the injectable drug ketamine, would be given first as the induction agent.

"They're here," Tom said, seeing the headlights outside the window.

"Okay, just a few more things and we're almost ready," I said. I took out a couple bottles of IV dextrose solution and some catheter equipment and moved the EKG machine and surgical light stand into place.

We were soon all assembled in the prep room, and it would be a first for all of us. Dr. Linda Albion was an OB/GYN professor at the university's medical school. She had delivered plenty of humans but never a gorilla. Dr. Arthur "Kip" Kipper was a university hospital professor in anesthesiology and was looking forward to the opportunity of passing gas to a gorilla for the first time in his career. The neonatologist was a university hospital pediatrician by the name of Dr. Betsy Jenkins, who had been handed hundreds of newborns following Caesarean section operations but never an infant primate. I would be the assistant surgeon and Tom would be the scrub nurse.

When Tom and I entered Lulu's cage I could tell she was a bit woozy from the Ativan. Tom took both of her hands in his and explained to Lulu what was going to happen next. "We need to give you an injection but I don't want you to worry, everything will be okay," Tom said to her. "Ready, here we go, girl." He looked at me and nodded. I took the needle off the syringe of ketamine and lightly tapped Lulu's tush while counting one, two, and three. "Good job, Tom, she never flinched," I said after I had attached the 12 cc syringe and pushed.

Within ten minutes Lulu was out cold. It took all five of us to move her onto the gurney and wheel her over to where we had set up our temporary surgery suite.

Dr. Kipper got an IV catheter going, hooked Lulu up to some fluids, and commented on Lulu's breath and large fang-like canine teeth while inserting an endotracheal tube into her windpipe. Tom shaved and scrubbed up her pregnant belly with some betadine disinfect and alcohol while I attached Lulu to the EKG and blood pressure monitor. Dr. Albion set up her surgery tray and Dr. Jenkins adjusted the incubator and bassinet and arranged suction cords and tubes to clear the baby's mouth once it was born.

Lulu's belly was clipped, prepped, and draped. Her endotracheal tube was attached to a ventilator and a triple gas anesthetic cocktail had her in a state of general anesthesia. An IV with fluids was running, and even though we didn't know the normal blood pressure values for a gorilla, we were monitoring her BP readings to ensure they remained fairly constant throughout the surgery. The screen of the EKG machine was beeping a steady rate and rhythm and with that, Dr. Albion asked, "Are we set to go?"

"She's good on my end," Dr. Kipper replied, making some fine adjustments on the gas anesthetic mix. "Are we taking bets on a boy or girl?" Dr. Jenkins commented while slipping on her sterile gloves.

"I don't know about a girl or boy but I've been thinking about a name I'm gonna suggest to the zoo director," Tom replied.

"Don't tell us now, Tom," I interrupted. "Let's wait to make sure everything goes okay."

Not too many gorilla C-sections had been done before in the United States but there we were at almost 2:00 A.M., the five of us gathered over Lulu in the prep room of the primate house, ready to begin.

Dr. Albion gave us a running discourse on what she was

doing from the moment she picked up the scalpel blade. We listened and watched as she talked about making a low transverse skin incision across Lulu's belly, retracting the skin and subcutaneous tissue, and then isolating and retracting the fascia that surrounds the *rectus abdominis*, one of the muscles of the belly. I helped control bleeding with hemostats, clamps, and gauze pads while she went on about the approach to the peritoneal cavity, emphasizing the need to incise superiorly to avoid the bladder. She then made another low transverse incision into the uterus, through the placental membranes to free up the head and umbilical cord of the baby.

"All right, all right, not too much traction on the cord," Dr. Jenkins said. "Let me get in there." She carefully lifted the baby gorilla out of the uterus and suctioned out the baby's mouth and airway. "Hmmm . . . good tone and movement," she declared.

It was another first for all of us, the cry of a newborn baby gorilla. Dr. Jenkins clamped the cord and placed the baby in the incubator while Dr. Albion began the hour-long procedure of suturing Lulu's incisions back together.

The anesthesiologist Dr. Virginia Apgar would likely have smiled that her "Apgar Score," which she developed in 1952 to assess the wellness of newborn humans, would one day also be used on an infant primate. Dr. Jenkins spent several minutes conducting her neonatal exam and assured us that Lulu's baby was a very healthy five-pound male.

We had anticipated there might be a different problem with Lulu's baby: Lulu rejecting it. Maternal behavior isn't an instinctual trait encrypted on one of the twenty-four pairs of the ape's chromosomes but rather is learned from watching other gorilla mothers bear and raise their young, an opportunity gorillas raised in captivity are for the most part deprived from experiencing. Other zoos, including the San Diego Zoo and the Bronx Zoo, had warned us of the likelihood that Lulu would perhaps want little if anything to do with her baby and that we should be prepared to raise it as an orphan.

Tom, however, had done some reading up on the learned maternal behavior of gorillas during Lulu's last couple months of gestation and had an idea. It was an idea that Tom's wife, Karen, initially thought to be somewhat odd but she was willing to give it a try. Tom and Karen had in the past year become parents themselves, and it was Tom's idea to have Karen visit him after work several times a week with their newborn infant and spend a few minutes outside Lulu's bedroom cage door.

During each of these many parenting sessions, Lulu was fascinated if not mesmerized when Karen coddled and held her baby. In Lulu's last few weeks of gestation, Karen had come up with an idea of her own. She stopped off at the toy store one afternoon on her way to the zoo to buy Lulu a baby doll which she would give to her in hopes that Lulu would mimic Karen's maternal care of her own baby. Time would tell.

"I wouldn't go in there without this," Tom said, handing me a broom. It was the next day and I was about to enter the rhino stockade with a glove and small plastic bag. I was back at the zoo to check on Lulu and her baby but also to examine Dino, one of the zoo's several black rhinos that had suddenly developed diarrhea.

"What's the broom for?" I asked Tom "All I need is a fecal sample to run some tests."

"You're kidding. You think you can just walk in and get

a fecal sample from a rhino?" Tom replied, shaking his head in disbelief at what I was about to do. "They're born mean and don't like strangers," Tom explained.

"Do you see that big pile over there?" he asked, pointing to what looked like a small hill in the middle of the enclosure. "That's the communal dung heap and that's where Dino is gonna drag you after he's shishkabobbed you a new one if you try and go up behind him with a silly glove and a plastic bag," Tom exclaimed.

"I didn't know that rhinos are aggressive," I remarked. "They're herbivores. They like to eat grass and browse around."

"Is that all they taught you about rhinos in vet school?" Tom asked, taking the broom back from me. "You better let me do this," he said. "How big a sample do you need?"

"Not much, a teaspoon-size amount of manure would be plenty," I answered, handing him the latex glove and small plastic bag.

As Tom entered the rhino stockade armed with the long-handled bristle broom, Dino turned to have a look from the other side of the dung heap and then put his head down with his three-foot-long horn menacingly aimed toward Tom. "I bet they didn't teach you that a rhino can charge at thirty-five miles an hour," Tom shouted back at me.

"You're right. I didn't know that," I yelled back from the other side of the stockade.

"Did they mention that when a rhino is feeling extra mean they'll charge a tree trunk just because, or that 50 percent of rhinos in the wild die from combat-related injuries? Did they teach you that?" Tom shouted.

"Nope, they never taught us that either," I yelled back. I could see Tom shaking his head at how little I knew about the aggressive nature of rhinos while muttering sarcastically something about how they liked to eat grass and browse around.

From the other side of the dung heap Dino stared at Tom, who was waving the broom back and forth, then he suddenly broke into a trot toward Tom. "Hey, Tom, maybe you better get outta there," I shouted.

Head down and horn up, the rhino's pace was quickening, and I imagined what would happen next. He would charge like some crazed bull lining up a matador in the crosshairs of his horns, and I was about to witness the impaling of a zookeeper by a black rhino.

Remarkably, the two-horned, three-thousand-pound black rhino came to a sudden halt only a few feet in front of Tom. It was then that Tom extended the broom under Dino's belly and began to rub. The rhino's eyes closed and his legs began to buckle out from underneath him. "Works every time," Tom said, vigorously brooming the rhino's underbelly.

As Dino lay on his side and Tom continued to scratch his belly with the broom, a thunderous flatus was expelled through the rhino's anus. A thirty-or-so-gallon diarrheic event shortly followed the impressive blowout, and the fetid smell reached me where I stood. "How much did you say you needed?" Tom shouted back at me, smiling.

The Rhinocerotidae demonstrate their affinity with the Equidae in the similarity of internal parasites each hosts. Genera common to both families include several nematodes such as *Anoplocephala* (tapeworms), *Oxyuris* (pinworms), and *Strongylus* (bloodworms).

A microscopic exam of Dino's manure revealed a heavy parasite load of an assortment of nematodes, including

Strongyloides, *Habronema*, *Oxyuris*, and *Kiluluma*, resulting in intestinal inflammation and diarrhea.

Fortunately for Dino, a recent and dramatic breakthrough in research by a pharmaceutical company by the name of Merck had just developed an anthelmintic, or dewormer, for humans to combat one of the leading causes of infectious blindness in the world. The parasitic disease onchocerciasis, or river blindness, is a devastating infection of humans and is endemic in thirty-seven countries in both Africa and Latin America.

Merck was well aware that an array of lifesaving drugs are produced by fungi, including the antibiotic penicillin, and they were about to add another to the list.

In its endeavor to find a cure for river blindness, Merck stumbled upon a remarkable chemical-producing fungus first isolated from soil samples obtained from a Japanese golf course. The compound produced by the fungus was unique for two reasons: The fungal metabolite not only had an unusual affinity to bind to the membranes of neurons of parasites such as nematodes and arthropods, but it also had the capacity to disrupt their nerve impulses.

The dewormer that would save millions of people from losing their sight to a parasitic microfilaria was the metabolite of a fungus having the unique neurotoxic capability of destroying the parasite without harming the mammalian host. The new wonder drug would be called Ivermectin.

In just a few years the silver bullet anthelmintic Ivermectin would become the most effective dewormer to be used not only in humans but in any number of other species, including guinea pigs, primates, camels, cattle, swine, horses, and of course rhinos.

"He's gonna need a couple glug-glugs of this," I said to

Tom as I poured several ounces of Ivermectin over Dino's ten-pound daily ration of apples, pears, and carrots.

"You think we should do the same with the other six rhinos?" Tom asked.

"Without a doubt if Dino is packing a heavy parasite load the others are too," I responded and began to measure out more doses to pour over each of the remaining six ten-pound buckets of fruit and vegetables.

"Rwanda, have you ever been there?" Tom asked me as we headed over to the gorilla house.

"Why would I want to go to a country entrenched in civil war and strife?" I asked.

"You should go. They have a lot of gorillas there and besides, people should be more concerned about what goes on in Africa," Tom said. "The director liked it and so did Doc Jenkins."

"What did they like about it?" I asked.

"The name," Tom replied as we opened the door to the gorilla house and stepped into the footbath.

"What are you talking about?" I asked.

"The name of course, the name I came up with for Lulu's baby: Rwanda."

Dr. Jenkins, the neonatologist, had remained throughout the early morning hours with Rwanda after Lulu's Caesarean section. Lulu had since been moved from the makeshift surgery suite in the prep room to an improvised post-op recovery room—her bedroom—which we had heavily bedded with straw. Lulu was awake but still a bit woozy from the general anesthetic, and Dr. Jenkins felt that the time had come and that Tom should be the one . . .

It was a gathering of silent skeptics. We were all somewhat anxious about what would happen next. Looming in our midst was the admonition from other zoos that Rwanda would likely be rejected by Lulu and that we should be prepared to bottle-feed an orphaned gorilla for the next three years.

Lulu had been fascinated and probably entertained by the parenting sessions made up of Tom's wife Karen nurturing and coddling their own newborn infant outside Lulu's cage. Yet other than Tom, no one actually believed that Karen's attempt to model out parenting skills for Lulu could possibly amount to anything more than a sort of primate-time TV.

The director of the zoo, myself, and several other zookeepers had gathered for the occasion. We watched Dr. Jenkins lift Rwanda from the open warmer incubator and pass him to Tom. Tom made his way over to Lulu's cage with Rwanda and opened the door. Lulu, still a little groggy, sat up from her bed of straw as Tom approached her. "I didn't think you'd mind if I came up with a name for him so I did," Tom said, kneeling down in front of her holding Rwanda in his arms.

"His name is Rwanda and he's getting hungry," Tom continued as he leaned toward Lulu, showing her what he had cradled in his arms. "He's gonna need you to take care of him and I know you'll be a great mom," Tom added as Lulu stared silently at little Rwanda for a few moments before looking back up at Tom.

"All right, Lulu, you have to take him now. He's needing to nurse," Tom said. He gently placed Rwanda at Lulu's chest.

Little Rwanda was like other gorilla infants, who have the ability shortly after birth to cling to their mother's chest with a very powerful grip from their hands and feet. Rwanda knew just what to do. He clasped on to Lulu's chest.

Tom helped support little Rwanda close to Lulu's chest and waited. All of us in the room were still and also waiting to see what would follow. It was then that Rwanda let out a little whimper and with that it happened. Lulu looked down at him, reached up with her powerful long arm, and pressed him to her chest.

Gorilla infants grow and develop much quicker than human babies. They begin playing, smiling, and bouncing around at eight weeks, crawling a week or so later, and walking by six months. Before the end of my year-long internship, Tom and I were among the first to see little Rwanda figure out how to climb on his mother's back and ride.

Lulu and Rwanda became one of the zoo's biggest attractions over the next months, and it was Tom who quietly took the greatest pride in knowing that the gorilla house was what everyone crowded to see. Rwanda's antics brought endless smiles, and "Oh, how cute" seemed to be heard the most amidst the "Oooohs" and "Ahhhs."

It was a Saturday morning and I was at the veterinary school, finishing up a case with some senior students on a foal that had been sent in with pneumonia, when I was paged by the large-animal clinic's secretary. "Tom at the zoo called. He said they have a pretty big problem at the Thai Village, something about Babar, and they need your help right away."

"Did he say anything more?" I asked.

"Nope, that was it. He sounded in a hurry and I told him I'd have you over there within the hour," she said.

The Thai Village was a part of the zoo that included an assortment of exhibits and habitats featuring animals from Asia. I chuckled to myself driving to the zoo recalling the message Tom left with the clinic's secretary. He knew I would catch his subtle humor in the message about a "pretty big problem."

Babar weighed almost eight thousand pounds. He was a fourteen-year-old Indian bull elephant, a circus retiree trained to ride a tricycle, and he had performed for several years before he became too difficult to manage at the young age of five. He was unchained and free now, living, roaming, and luxuriating in the zoo's forest habitat, which included enormous rock formations with ponds and waterfalls.

Babar was never "too difficult to manage," as the circus claimed, he just didn't like riding tricycles. For a bull elephant he was in fact pretty much of a big cupcake with a giant-size sense of humor.

An elephant's trunk is remarkably versatile and Babar used his elongated appendage or proboscis to lift, greet, caress, and also as a snorkel when the rest of him disappeared underwater in the elephant lake. Over the course of a day Babar used his trunk to wrap around about three hundred pounds of hay and stuff it into his mouth. And it was his trunk that greeted me much like a handshake whenever he saw me and with the fingerlike projections from the tip of his trunk daintily managed to grasp one by one his favorite snack from the palm of my hand: cranberries.

Elephants also use their trunks to drink by sucking up three to four gallons of water at a time and blowing it into their mouths or to spray water over their backs as sort of an anywhere shower and to cool themselves off, as elephants don't have the ability to sweat.

The elephant is a symbol of wisdom in Asian cultures and famed for its memory, intelligence, and at times, I might add, humor. Elephants had Super Soakers long before kids did, and when Babar drew up a trunkful of water, one was never quite sure of his intentions. If you splashed him first, a return soaking volley was pretty much a sure thing. If it was a hot summer's day, he'd cool himself down, but if on occasion he was feeling a bit naughty, it might be an unsuspecting Thai Village visitor that received a drenching spray.

I drove through the gates of the Thai Village and headed over to the elephant habitat, where I could see Tom waiting for me. "Hey, Tom, what's going on with Babar?" I asked.

"Thanks for coming so quick. I'm not sure," Tom replied. "He came up lame on his right front foot pretty much just all of a sudden and he's got a bunch of pus coming out from one of his toes."

"C'mon, let's go have a look," I said.

"Hang on a sec, be right back. I forgot something," I said to Tom as we were about to enter the elephant stockade. I dashed back to my vet truck, opened the glove box, and grabbed the Ocean Spray bag.

"Elephants never forget, and he'd never forgive you if you forgot those," Tom remarked smiling at seeing what I had in my hand when I returned.

"Hey, big guy, what's going on? Look what I've got," I said holding out a handful of cranberries. Babar gently wrapped his trunk around my arm and began to pluck several cranberries from the palm of my hand. Tom was right, Babar was barely placing any weight on his right front foot and seeping from his outside toe was a thick and yellowish fetid exudate.

"There's a pretty nasty smell to that pus," I said, bending down to take a closer look at Babar's toe.

Despite their huge size and immense weight, elephants walk on their toes, perhaps something akin to an eight-thousand-pound ballerina but without the tutu. Their legs become cylindrical at the level of their foot, and because their heels are slightly elevated, the five digits in the forefeet come down at a steep angle, predisposing them to any number of foot problems.

I knelt down with a handful of gauze pads and a squirt bottle of soapy iodine disinfect and cleaned Babar's big toe. It was not his big toe in the sense of being the *biggest* toe, in the way a person has a small, bit bigger, big, even bigger, and biggest toe, but more in the sense that even though an elephant's five toes are all the same size, they're all still big.

"Have a look, Tom, check this out," I said, pointing to a black fistulous tract in Babar's toenail. It was a dissecting fissure in the toenail tunneling back to the cuticle, from which the purulent exudate was oozing.

"What is it?" Tom asked as I probed the infected draining tract.

"He's got a nasty toe abscess that extends pretty deep into the foot that could even be brewing into a phalangeal osteomyelitis," I told him.

"A what?" Tom asked.

"A bone infection in his foot" I replied. "We're gonna have to shoot some films but first I need to take a culture and sensitivity."

I inserted a six-inch sterile cotton swab into the draining tract. "That goes in pretty deep and I'm up against bone," I said to Tom. "This will tell us what type of bacteria is involved and which antibiotic to treat him with." I withdrew the swab and placed it into a tube containing culture media to take back to the lab. "I'll be right back. Let me get the portable X-ray machine and some plates out the back of the truck and we'll take some films." I headed back to my vet truck.

I returned with the portable radiograph machine I used on the legs of horses and a couple of lead aprons and several cassette plates. "Here's the game plan," I said to Tom, helping him snug up the straps of his lead apron. "We'll take some films and then poultice up his foot with a drawing salve. It'll take a couple days for the culture to come back from the lab but in the meantime I'll at least have a chance to look at the X-ray films later today and have some idea how serious the infection is."

Babar's massive triple E–size foot would require cranking up all the settings on my portable X-ray machine well beyond what I would ever use on even the biggest draft horse foot. I would also have to take several views of the foot from different angles and directions to be able to accurately image the phalanx, or bony digit, of the affected toe to rule in or out an osteomyelitis.

"Okay, Tom, just a couple more and we'll be done," I remarked. I had taken a lateral view, several obliques, and was kneeling down holding the X-ray machine as still as possible to take an A-P, or anterior-posterior view, when I felt something warm tickling and blowing on my neck. "Hold on a sec," I said to Tom, putting down the X-ray machine and standing up.

"Okay Babar, but no more after this," I said, reaching into my back pocket for the bag of Ocean Spray.

"That should keep him quiet till we're done," I said to Tom and knelt back down, repositioning the X-ray machine.

The room was dark apart from the fluorescent light from the viewing screen. I had just finished putting the films up on the wall-mounted monitor when Dr. Cantrell, one of the radiology professors, walked in and asked, "Whadda ya got?"

I gave him the clinical history of Babar's lameness while

he scanned the films I had arranged on the viewing screen. "Should've burned these a little hotter," he remarked, referring to a couple of underexposed radiographs. "With this one here you would've gotten better contrast and less blur if you turned down the kVp and upped the mAs. And these last two could have been much more diagnostic with less scatter radiation had you used a 400-speed film/screen combination," he concluded pedantically.

Apparently shooting in the dark described the films I shot, which was all that the radiologist could see. I was familiar with the adjustable kVp (kilovolt peak) and the mAs (milliamp seconds) exposure settings on my portable X-ray machine when it came to horses, but I was left to improvise with Babar.

I felt discouraged and at least somewhat deserving of a "Nice try" or perhaps a "Good effort." After all, it was the first elephant's toe I had ever radiographed and besides, at the time of my internship the veterinary literature wasn't brimming with how-to's when it came to elephants.

"Well, is there anything at all diagnostic about the films?" I asked hopefully.

"Hmmm . . . they're not the best images," he reminded me, "but let's see. . . There's clearly some spiculated new bone growth as part of a periosteal reaction in the cortex of the distal aspect of the third phalanx. And if you look here, there's some endosteal scalloping at the corticomedullary junction and loss of trabecular architecture in the phalanx as well," he explained, pointing to the lesions. "There's more" he added. "The osteolytic changes occurring in the digit make it difficult to marginate portions of the distal phalanx. And that's pretty much it," he concluded, standing up to leave.

"Thanks so much, Dr. Cantrell. I really appreciate your

having a look," I responded.

"You're welcome," he answered, heading out the door.

"Um . . . Dr. Cantrell, wait before you go . . . S-so you think . . . ," I stammered and paused, hoping for somewhat more of a clinical interpretation of his findings.

University professors enjoy the status of their position and on occasion find ways in which they can subtly remind themselves of all they have achieved and accomplished. Here was just such an opportunity, the lowly intern at the feet of the full professor, an *amuse-bouche* if you will, from the French, similar to but not to be confused with an *hors d'oeuvre*, a tidbit, often tiny, served to keep one happy while waiting for the first course to come.

Basking loftily and relishing the moment, Dr. Cantrell was about to toss the dog a bone.

"Radiographically, I would conclude that even with the quality of these films being considerably less than ideal, your patient has a subacute osteomyelitis of his third phalanx," he remarked as he walked out the door.

I was back at the zoo the following day, changing the poulticed foot bandage on Babar with Tom, when an urgent message came through on his two-way radio. "C'mon hurry, it's Stretch—she's in labor. We gotta go," Tom told me just as I finished duct-taping Babar's foot.

The rising mist and audible roar that can be seen and heard for miles inspired the name given by Africans to the world's largest and most magnificent waterfall: the Smoke that Thunders.

The Victoria Falls are in central Africa, where the 2,200-mile Zambezi River leaves Zambia and flows into Zimbabwe. It was along the banks of the upper Zambezi that Stretch was born, a part of the continent where a wondrous array of African wildlife can be found.

Stretch was in the "Banks of the Zambezi River" exhibit that featured animals living along the spectacular river. There were hippos, zebras, crocodiles, hyenas, lions, the beautifully elegant and graceful yellow-billed storks, and Stretch and her mate Highto, both giraffes.

Stretch had been moved to an isolated area of the exhibit for the last two months of her fourteen-month pregnancy, a maternity leave of sorts from visitors, so as to be able to give birth to her calf peacefully and undisturbed.

It was no tall tale that Tom and I arrived in short order to see Stretch just as her baby was about to be born. "I got a name already," Tom told me in a hushed tone.

"Don't we need to wait to see if it's a boy or girl first?" I whispered.

"It doesn't matter and besides, the director liked it too," he replied as we watched the first placental sac appear.

Giraffes are timid, quiet animals, sort of like very tall cows without a moo. They're ruminants, having four stomachs, and chew their cud, which is to say that they swallow and regurgitate their food to chew it again.

Stretch was about twenty feet tall and weighed close on fourteen hundred pounds. Her coat was reticulated, consisting of liver-colored polygonal spots outlined by a network of bright white lines, like giant puzzle pieces. Her eyes seemed almost too big for her head . . . ah . . . but of course, the better to see with.

Giraffes are good to hang out with, especially if you are a zebra, antelope, or wildebeest and live along the banks of the Zambezi where lions come to stalk their next meal. Giraffes can see an enemy before its friends can and provide the early-warning mealtime alert.

It was bigger than just a *kerplunk,* Leggy's rather abrupt and startling entry into the world began with about an eight-foot free fall to earth. Giraffes give birth standing up. The cord breaks during descent, and ground impact is somewhat similar to the spank that a newborn baby receives to startle it to breathe for the first time.

Tom and I waited twenty minutes or so for Stretch to pass her placenta and Leggy to stand, before going to see if the calf was a male or female.

The tongue of a giraffe is almost two feet long and as prehensile as the tail of a monkey. They use their tongues to deftly grasp their favorite leafy food amidst the thorny branches of the acacia and mimosa trees but also to lick and groom their newborn calves.

"C'mon, she just passed her placenta. Let's go have a look," I said to Tom.

Leggy was the first giraffe calf I had ever seen born and like most newborn giraffes was able to stand within minutes after birth. "It's a bull calf," I said to Tom, thinking how odd it was to walk up to a newborn anything and have it be six feet tall, taller than the veterinarian trying to examine it.

Along the banks of the Zambezi River in central Africa, hungry crocodiles, packs of spotted hyenas, and stalking lions prey upon newborn giraffes, taking out more than half of the calves born every year. Leggy, on the other hand, would live to walk tall for twenty-five years or more among his Zambezi River companions, the hippos, the zebras, and antelope in the safety of the zoo.

There isn't much in the way of movie theaters or drive-ins in central Africa, but that doesn't stop giraffes from necking, a behavior somewhat different from what you might think. Dueling male giraffes, using their necks as weapons, swing their necks at each other in an attempt to land powerful blows to establish dominance, thus earning the right to court the likes of a Stretch.

"Any results back yet on Babar's culture and sensitivity?" I asked the lab tech when I stopped by the clinical pathology lab the following day.

"Hang on a sec, let me check," she responded.

University veterinary hospitals are set up very much like human hospitals in that they have their own departments of radiology, clinical pathology, surgery, and medicine. Veterinary schools also have their own pharmacies, which are different from those of human hospitals in that veterinary pharmacists must be somewhat creatively skilled in compounding medications to treat cats, dogs, horses, pet rabbits, and birds, not to mention the likes of reptiles, including iguanas and snakes, and giant mammals such as elephants.

"Gram-negative anaerobe, heavy growth *Bacteroides fragilis*" was what the culture and sensitivity report stated. The susceptibility pattern included several antibiotics, including chloramphenicol, a type of penicillin known as amoxicillin, clindamycin, lincomycin, and metronidazole.

I was relieved when I read the report, knowing that we would be able to effectively treat Babar's bone infection, but I also found myself smiling at the task Tom had before him.

"When do you think you'll have the prescription ready?" I asked the pharmacist.

"It's gonna take a while to make this up," he answered. "Probably sometime tomorrow afternoon. You want me to write dosage instructions on the script or are you gonna tell him?" the pharmacist asked, smiling at me.

"I better tell him," I responded.

I knew more about medicating elephants than I did about the aggressive nature of rhinos when formulating with the pharmacist the antibiotic I would need to treat Babar.

Babar had a serious infection, an osteomyelitis, that would require accurate and effective therapeutic dosing. Although mixing medications with food is easy, elephants are notorious for refusing oral medications and besides, there is almost always spillage and separation when trying to medicate their food. Additionally, because the drinking water of elephants is sometimes sprayed into their mouths and other times used to shower, soak, and splash themselves or others, administering drugs in their water isn't an accurate and effective means of medicating a sick elephant either.

Injections using jumbo-size syringes and needles are occasionally used but despite their large size and thick skin elephants are surprisingly sensitive to injections. Babar would need to be treated for a minimum of three weeks, and twice-daily big-needle injections of large volumes of an antibiotic for this length of time wouldn't be tolerated.

Of the list of antibiotics that the bacterial organism *Bacteroides fragilis* was sensitive to, metronidazole at a dose of 5 mg per pound of body weight administered once daily would be most effective. Doing the math meant that Babar, an eight-thousand-pound elephant, would require 40,000 mg of metronidazole to be administered daily.

Metronidazole is a highly effective oral antibiotic used in horses, but because of its bitter taste, horses are reluctant to eat their grain when this medication is added to it.

Fortunately, in both horses and elephants their rectal mucosa has an absorptive capability similar to that of their upper gastrointestinal tract. A single daily rectal administration of the antibiotic is equally as effective as oral dosing in achieving therapeutic plasma levels.

"Here ya go," the pharmacist said, handing me a box of elephant-size suppositories. "Your zookeeper friend is gonna need these as well," he added, giving me a three-week supply of shoulder-length sleeves and several squirt bottles of lube. "I guess the only other item missing from the prescription is a ladder," the pharmacist chuckled.

"Hey, Tom, I'm on my way with everything we need to treat Babar. I'll meet you at the Thai Village in an hour," I said. "Tom, wait, you still there? I almost forgot: We're gonna need a ladder," I added quickly, hanging up before he had a chance to ask why.

I headed off to the zoo, needing to make one more stop—the grocery store. Despite Babar's cupcake demeanor and giant-size sense of humor, Tom was still going to need a lot of cranberries.

Tom was waiting for me when I pulled up outside the elephant stockade in the Thai Village. Lying on the ground next to him was a ladder. "Good news: Babar is gonna be fine," I said.

"That's a relief. I was beginning to worry. So how we gonna treat him?" Tom asked.

"Here, take this," I said, handing Tom the box of Babar's medication but leaving the bag of sleeves and squirt bottles of lube behind the truck seat.

"Wow, these are the biggest gelatin capsules I've ever seen. How are we gonna get him to swallow these?" Tom asked.

The Bengal tiger is the national animal of both India and Bangladesh. It is also on the critically endangered list, in great part because of its perceived value in traditional

Chinese medicine.

Age-old doctrines of Chinese medicine are rooted in books such as the *Yellow Emperor's Inner Canon*, where seemingly scripted in stone for China's modern masses is the belief that there is near mystical healing power in almost all anatomical parts of the tiger.

Tiger bone cures dysentery, tiger claw is used to treat insomnia, its teeth have antipyretic or fever-reducing powers, tiger bile relieves convulsions in children, parts of a tiger's eye are of therapeutic value in treating epilepsy, and the fat of a tiger is one of the only cures for leprosy. Tiger whiskers will relieve a toothache and stated emphatically in Chinese medical texts is the only hope for alcoholism: tiger dung. Tragic but true is the fact that this hunter is hunted because purée of its brain is believed to offer up the cure for both laziness and acne, and its tail is as much an aphrodisiac as the horn of the rhinoceros. Sadly, today's Chinese medical practices, still steeped in myth and fallacy, have driven both tiger and rhino to the edge of extinction.

Several senior veterinary students and I were working up a lame Standardbred racehorse on a Friday morning when I was paged by the large-animal clinic's secretary. "It's Tom, he's worried about one of the tigers and hopes you can take a look before the weekend."

I was back at the Thai Village that afternoon and drove to the tiger exhibit, where I saw Tom waiting for me. For just a moment of pause and reflection as I parked my vet truck, giving Tom a wave, I was saddened by the thought of my year-long internship coming to an end. My original large-animal internship plans—not to be distracted by the likes of cats or dogs but rather to pursue what nickers and neighs—had taken somewhat of a serendipitous detour. Humor, respect, fun, and a passion for the animals at the zoo had provided an opportunity for Tom and me to become close friends. There was a knowing of sorts that we both shared about the privilege of working with such strange and marvelous animals.

I climbed out of my truck. "Hey, Tom, what's going on?" I asked.

"It's Bengali, he busted off his lower right canine a couple of weeks ago. I didn't think it was going to be a problem but he seems cranky lately, not eating well and batting his face with his paw every once in a while like it's bothering him," Tom told me as we headed over to the fenced enclosure.

Bengali was a ten-year-old male Bengal tiger now safely living in the Columbus Zoo, having been rescued from Chinese poachers at the early age of four.

"He sure is a beauty," I remarked, admiring Bengali's coloring and markings as we stood outside his cage.

"He'd have you for lunch, you know," Tom commented, as if I didn't know anything about four-hundred-pound flesh-eating cats.

"That or drag me in and save me for later," I responded.

"Well, at least they taught you more about tigers than they did about rhinos in veterinary school," he added with a nudging elbow to my ribs.

It took a while before biologists understood the camouflaging strategy of the tiger's stripes. The preyed-upon meals of tigers are for the very most part other wild animals such as deer or antelope, which are color-blind. The about-to-be-eaten antelope sees the tiger's vertical stripes only as bands of shadow and light in the tall grass. The rest of the giant cat isn't actually seen by its next meal until it is altogether too late.

Bengali gave a growl and I could see that what Tom had said was true: Bengali's lower right canine had fractured off more than midway.

The killer four big fangs that a tiger uses to grab the throat of its prey are called canines, even though they have nothing to do with what barks. The upper two canines are what a dentist would call the maxillary cuspids and the lower two the mandibular cuspids. Each canine is ordinarily three to four inches in length, having a pulp cavity or canal, and is deeply rooted in the upper (maxilla) or lower (mandible) jawbones. A fractured canine is of concern because it exposes the root canal, allowing bacteria from the oral cavity access to the tooth root in the jawbone, invariably resulting in an osteomyelitis.

"What do you think? Leave it and do a wait and see?" Tom asked.

"I kinda don't think so," I responded. "That's a three- or four-inch tooth with a canal in the middle of it that he's fractured off."

"What's wrong in just waiting to see what happens?" Tom asked.

"Well, it's sort of like Babar's toe," I answered.

"Oh no, we're not doing that again," Tom was quick to reply.

"Not to worry, Bengali is probably gonna need some antibiotics but he'll take 'em in a hunk of meat," I said.

"It's a good thing you called," I told him. "He's cranky, not eating, and batting his face because he's likely already got a jawbone infection that's inflamed and hurting."

After a minute or so of watching the big cat and seeing him take a swipe at his jaw with his massive right front paw,

I said "You and I can't do this, Tom, we're going to need some help."

"Ever been to an endodontist?"

"A what?" Tom asked.

"If ever you'd been to one, you'd know what they do. They're pricey, painful, and it's never just one visit. They're a dentist but they do more . . . kinda like an orthodontist does braces but these guys do root canals."

"How you gonna get Bengali to say 'Ahhh' for the dentist?" Tom asked.

I consulted with the chief veterinarian of the large animal clinic and he advised me to head over to the dental school and see if I could find one of the clinicians to help us out. "And what about anesthesia?" I asked.

"I'll take care of that" he answered.

The College of Dentistry at Ohio State University is one of the largest in the country, having all of the subspecialties, including orthodontics, periodontics, oral and maxillofacial surgery, implant surgery, and endodontics. "I'm game," a professor in endodontics declared after I explained the dilemma of a tiger needing a root canal at the Columbus Zoo. "I'll bring a couple of residents along and make it a teaching opportunity," he added.

Tom had Bengali isolated in a separate cage by the time the rest of us arrived. There was the professor of endodontics from the dental school, two of his residents, the chief veterinarian of the large-animal clinic, myself, and Tom.

"Better stand back," the chief of the large-animal clinic instructed us as he removed from his grip syringes, needles, and vials of M99 and M5050. He wore gloves and goggles as he withdrew into a syringe dart less than one half a cc of the super-potent morphine-like drug M99. "You're a goner if this stuff gets on your skin or in your eyes," he warned us.

M99 (etorphine hydrochloride) is a super-potent opiate related to morphine but about ten thousand times stronger. It's a powerful, extremely fast acting immobilizing agent used to capture wild game. An injection of only a few drops can drop a rhino or an elephant in less than a minute. Veterinarians use it in zoos as do game wardens when they take aim at the hungry black bear that has wandered out of the woods into the neighborhood communities, tipping over garbage cans. Unfortunately, deluded and fueled by medical myth, Chinese tiger and rhino poaching syndicates also use it.

"Catatonia" is defined as a state of paralysis-like stupor and M99, once injected, makes it happen fast. "Catalepsy" is the medical term used to describe what happens next in the downed animal. Its posture becomes fixed in sort of a Gumby-like, waxy rigidity, so that their limbs remain in whatever position they are placed.

Once done with the downed and out, a fast-acting reversing agent is administered. Within minutes of injecting the rapidly acting opioid antagonist M5050 (Diprenorphine), the immobilized is remobilized.

From its protective case, the clinic chief removed a single bolt-action rifle and inserted the carbon dioxide propelled syringe dart into the chamber. Turning to me as he closed the breech bolt on the rifle, he said, "So, Doc, tell me about the pharmacology of M99."

I was only a year out of veterinary school, a lowly intern, a peon and plebe in the eyes of full professors and others with tenure, and was being quizzed by the head of the large-animal clinic in front of a small audience.

I had been diminished and belittled as a senior in

veterinary school, falling into the trap of the unprepared during rounds, when a small group of students and clinicians would gather outside a patient's stall. Professors would question the students regarding medications, laboratory results, and the nature of the illness, injury, or disease of the patient. Students with incorrect answers, "I'm not sures," and "I don't knows" were ready fodder for stallside inquisitions and verbal lynchings by irascible professors.

I had done some reading the night before. "Well, sir, it seems to me that I recall that M99 or to be more specific, etorphine hydrochloride, was first synthesized in 1963. It's a synthetic opioid related to morphine but much more potent. Its use in immobilizing game animals results largely from its ability to cause catatonia at very low dose levels. Typically, the muscular state of the immobilized animal is that of catalepsy," I responded, sensing that the barrel of the rifle was no longer pointed in my direction.

"So would you agree then that the anesthetic characteristics of both *cat*atonia and *cat*alepsy to be induced by M99 are appropriate for a tiger?" he then asked me.

"Yes sir," I replied, not realizing his academic attempt at humor.

"And what do you suppose of the outcome if I were to give the tiger more than the required dose?" he further questioned me.

"Well, sir, given the fact that M99 is extremely potent, an overdose would likely result in . . ."

"*Catacombs!*" he blurted out with a smile, glancing at us all.

Being that he was a professor and head of the large-animal clinic and the person from whom I would one day likely request a letter of recommendation, I was the first to applaud his insight and wit. "Oh, very good, sir, quite funny. I get it now . . . tiger, cat, catatonia, catalepsy, catacombs."

Tom and I managed to lift four hundred pounds of cat onto a portable table and set up some surgical lights while the dental team arranged their instruments.

Myself, Tom, and the head of the large-animal clinic peered as best we could over the shoulders of the dental trio as they discussed and strategized the endodontic challenge of Bengali's fractured canine. "There's approximately fifty millimeters of crown missing and the pulp cavity has significant decay," one of the residents remarked while exploring the hollows of the fractured cuspid.

"Irrigate as you excavate," the dental professor reminded his residents as they used an assortment of wires, drills, tiny files called endofiles, and irrigating solutions to remove the diseased nerves, blood vessels, and cellular debris from the pulp chamber. The dental professor supervised, instructed, and inspected the work of his residents as they completed the first stage of the procedure. "Ready to obturate?" the professor asked.

"Almost," responded one of the residents.

Removing or excavating the diseased tissue from the hollows of the pulp cavity is the first stage of a root canal surgery and obturation is the second. The word "obturate" means to fill or close, and obturation of the decontaminated pulp chamber is what's done next using a range of inert fillers, amalgams, cements, and sealers.

"That should do it," the dental professor exclaimed, turning to myself, Tom, and the head of the large-animal clinic.

Bengali had been down for almost two hours for the root canal surgery and had just been administered the reversing agent M5050. "It's done. We have three minutes to be out of his cage unless one of you wishes to join him for dinner," the head of the large-animal clinic said following the injection.

It was a couple of months later when I received a letter regarding my application to the equine residency program at the veterinary school in California. It seemed that a favorable letter of recommendation had been written by the head of the large-animal clinic on my behalf.

My year-long internship in Ohio came to an end in early June and I was expected to begin my residency a week later. I would leave for California a day later than I had planned. I spent that day at the zoo, as a visitor and not as a veterinarian, marveling at the array of the exotic and bizarre, the languid and the lumbering, the colorful and the curious, and laughing a few laughs with my good friend Tom.

Acknowledgements

I would very much like to acknowledge the wonderful help, encouragement and support of Della Mancuso who managed the entire project; Mary Kornblum for her terrific design of text and cover, incorporating the lovely painting and drawings by Susan Dorazio.